Half Marathon

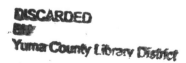

The contents of this book were carefully researched. However, all information is supplied without liability. Neither the authors nor the publisher will be liable for possible disadvantages or damages resulting from this book.

JEFF & BARBARA GALLOWAY

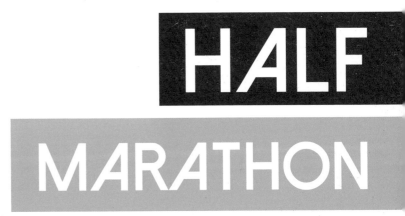

HALF
MARATHON

A COMPLETE TRAINING GUIDE FOR WOMEN

Meyer & Meyer Sport

British Library Cataloguing in Publication Data

A catalogue record for this book is available from the British Library

Half Marathon: A Complete Training Guide for Women

Maidenhead: Meyer & Meyer Sport (UK) Ltd., 2019

ISBN: 978-1-78255-164-5

© 2019 by Meyer & Meyer Sport (UK) Ltd.
2nd edition 2019 of the 1st edition 2012

Aachen, Auckland, Beirut, Cairo, Cape Town, Dubai, Hägendorf, Hong Kong, Indianapolis, Manila, New Delhi, Singapore, Sydney, Tehran, Vienna

 Member of the World Sport Publishers' Association (WSPA)

Manufacturing: Print Consult GmbH, Munich, Germany

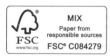

ISBN: 978-1-78255-164-5
Email: info@m-m-sports.com
www.m-m-sports.com

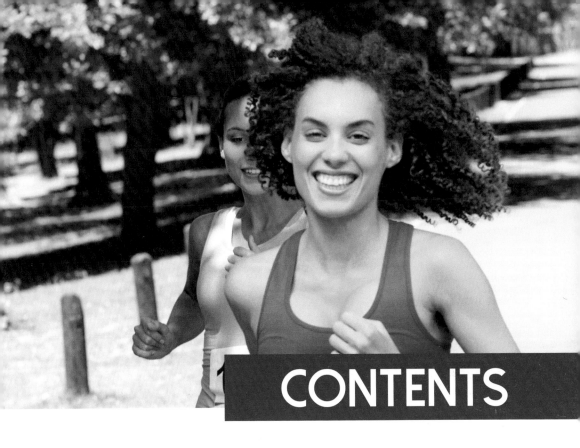

CONTENTS

INTRODUCTION: YOU CAN DO IT!

This book is dedicated to the approximately 3 million women who start training for a half marathon each year. Because of a number of issues, only about 20% make it to the finish line. It is our mission to reduce the dropout rate to almost zero by providing motivation, solutions to problems, injury-free training, and a two-hour-a-week training program during most weeks.

We are inspired to hear the stories from thousands each year who get off the couch and finish a half marathon. The empowerment from this accomplishment often results in taking more control over one's attitude. I hear stories every day about how the half marathon journey led to achievement and problem solving in other areas of life.

We look forward to hearing your story at an event, a beach retreat, or one of our many clinics throughout the US each year. If you have not taken on a challenging goal before, welcome to the positive, supportive, and inspiring community of runners. If you have done this before and want to improve, welcome back!

Barbara Galloway　　　　*Jeff Galloway*

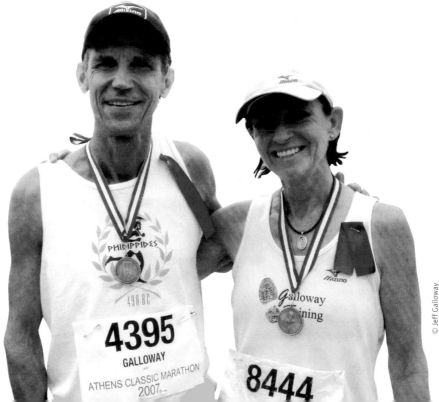

A NOTE TO WALKERS

The "to finish" schedule in this book has been used by tens of thousands of walkers to cross the half marathon finish line. The chapters on nutrition, motivation, women's issues, weather, etc. apply to walkers and runners. There is one training component that is different. Runners will take "walk breaks" to stop the continuous use of the orthopedic units that cause aches, pains, excess fatigue, burnout, and injury. Walkers have a variation that provides the same benefit: "shuffle breaks." Every 3-5 minutes, during a long walk, reduce your stride length for 30 seconds and let the feet, legs, hips, and back recover. During these breaks, focus on the enjoyment of exercise and positive thoughts.

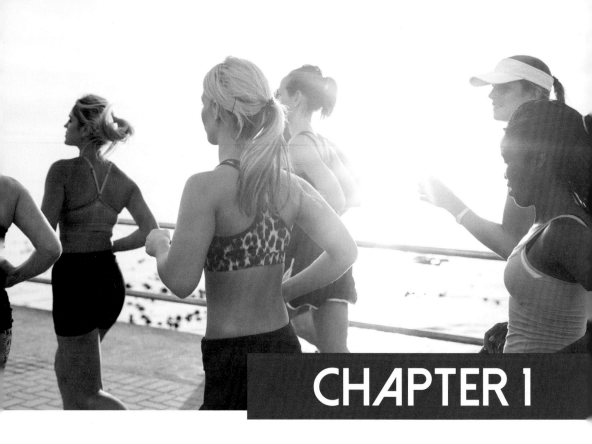

CHAPTER 1

WHY DO WOMEN LOVE
THE HALF MARATHON?

- One can train for a half marathon and carry on family/social/career activities
- The empowerment from a half marathon helps women confront other challenges
- The "mission" of the 13.1 distance gives meaning to each training run, improving motivation
- Each run can boost attitude, vitality and self-esteem, energizing the day
- Even after a difficult 13.1 mile (21K) race, runners can usually celebrate that evening
- Beginners who yearn to run a marathon see this distance as the first big step
- Marathoners find that the "half" keeps them in shape for their next "full"
- Using the Run-Walk-Run method in this book saves energy to carry on life activities
- Increasing long runs for a half marathon often results in faster times at 5K, 10K, etc.

- There are very few achievements in life as satisfying as training/finishing a half marathon

- Almost all of the concerns women have about running are addressed in this book and are usually not causes for concern

- Runners have healthier orthopedic units than non-runners as the years go by

Women are flooding into half marathons in record numbers. Surprisingly, many have never been active in sports or fitness activities. The experience is so positive that every finisher wants to tell others about the great benefits. The result: every half marathoner influences more than 20 people to either train for a half marathon or to add fitness to their lifestyle. Sisters pull sisters off the couch, and mothers influence children to be active. At women's events, such as the Jeff Galloway Half Marathon in Atlanta *(www.jeffgalloway131.com)*, there are non-stop stories of mother-daughter, college roommates, and long-term friends. They share the training journey (sometimes when living in different cities) and run the event together.

Women like to have control over their lives. Many of these newly addicted half marathoners tell me that it was my Run-Walk-Run method that induced them to sign up and train. You'll see later in the book how this method reduces aches, pains, injuries, and extra fatigue. Each woman decides how much to run and walk on a given day to remain in charge.

The role model effect of this surge in women in half marathons is exciting. Research shows that exercising mothers tend to have exercising kids. I've now heard thousands of stories from kids or adults who began their own fitness journey because they had a mom who finished a half marathon.

This is a totally doable training program for almost everyone. The minimal running time can be inserted into very busy lives. Enjoy every run and you will not only cross the 13.1 mile finish line: you're likely to be addicted for life.

There are worse addictions.

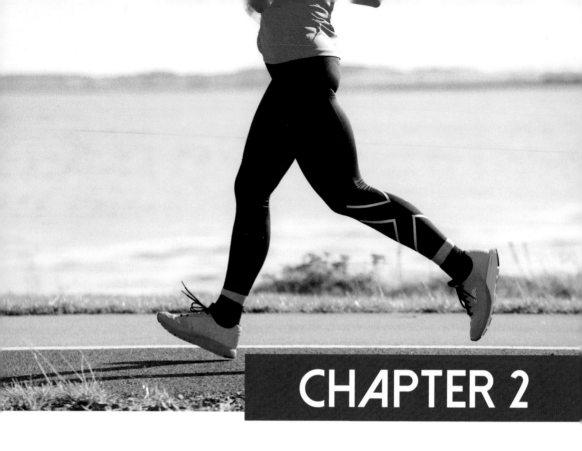

CHAPTER 2

READ THIS FIRST (TO STAY INJURY-FREE)

GOOD NEWS AND BAD NEWS ABOUT WOMEN AND INJURIES

Good News: Women tend to follow conservative guidelines in training. When they stay below the threshold of pain, the injury rate and lingering fatigue is near zero.

Bad News: When women don't follow the conservative guidelines, such as those in this book, they experience more injuries and a longer recovery time. Primary causes are not having a good training schedule, increasing the duration or speed of training too quickly, running the long runs too fast, or failing to use the conservative Run-Walk-Run strategy for the current level of conditioning.

By focusing on certain key principles, and running with them, it's possible to do a half marathon and carry on family, social, career activities without pain or sustained tiredness.

- You have control over pace. Always choose a slower pace, especially during long runs or any run when you are feeling your "weak links." If you slow down on the long runs, you'll receive the same endurance while reducing the recovery time. Specific pace guidelines are included in this book.

- Take liberal walk breaks on long runs. You will experience the same endurance whether you run 10 seconds every minute or run 10 minutes and walk one minute. When in doubt, ease back into more walking and less running. Walk break guidelines are included in this book.

- Your body is programmed to heal itself if you let it. Ease off on any workout if you feel any aches, pains, huffing, or problem of concern. Even running for a few minutes, when you have incurred an injury, can greatly increase the damage and the healing period.

- Begin your training at your current level – don't jump ahead because a friend is running that distance. If you are behind on a schedule for an event, you can "make up the distance" by gently walking at the beginning of the next long run for the distance you need to catch up.

- Gradually increase! Increasing distance too quickly (long run or weekly mileage) is a major cause of aches, pains, and excess fatigue. Increasing speed repetitions too quickly can also lead to injury.

- Running every other day significantly reduces injury risk. This allows the body to rebuild and improve after each workout.

- If you increase the amount of running vs. walking on short runs, do it gradually.

- First time 13.1 trainees: don't do speedwork and don't shoot for a time goal.

- Veterans should ease into speed training. It is too easy for an experienced runner to push too hard in the beginning of a speed training program and become injured, chronically fatigued, or burned out and frustrated. Let the body gradually adapt.

- At the first sign of a possible injury, stop the run and take at least two days off from running. If you allow the healing to begin, you may be able to continue running while the healing continues.

- Stay below the threshold of irritation. Most of the runners who have come to me when injured have been able to continue running when they slowed the pace and inserted walk breaks frequently enough to avoid further irritation.

- Don't let men lead you astray! Men have greater bone density and tougher muscle and tendon connections than women. If you are having aches and pains when trying to keep up with a spouse or male running buddy, back off immediately.

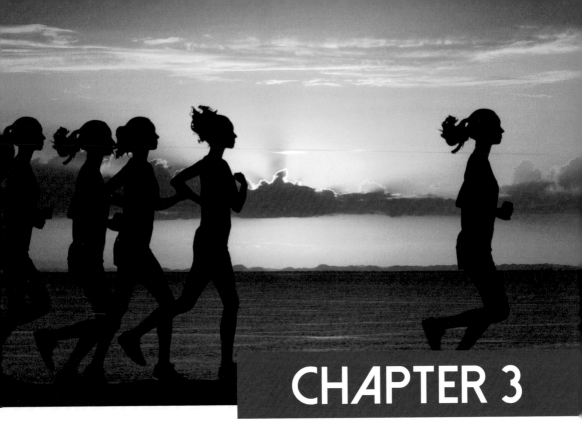

CHAPTER 3

SETTING GOALS AND PRIORITIES

By focusing on a few key elements, you have the opportunity to take control over the enjoyment of the running experience. If you're preparing for your first half marathon race, I recommend that you choose the "to finish" schedule, and run slower on every run than you could run on that day. Even after the 20th or 100th race, you're more likely to remember the details of your first one.

Your mission, therefore, should be to weave the training runs, and the race itself, into a positive tapestry of memories that will enrich the rest of your life.

TOP THREE GOALS (EVEN FOR TIME-GOAL RUNNERS)

1. Finish in the upright position,

2. with a smile on your face,

3. wanting to do it again.

These three components define the primary level of success in any training program, and the degree of enjoyment of each long run. If this is your first race experience at the 13.1 distance, visualize yourself coming across the finish line, demonstrating these three behaviors. The more you focus on this image, the more likely you are to follow the guidelines and experience this during most of your runs.

RUNNING ENJOYMENT

Find a way to enjoy parts of every run – even the speed training (if you are a time-goal runner). Most of your runs should be mostly enjoyable. You increase the pleasure of each run by inserting a few social/scenic/mentally refreshing runs every week.

Your desire to take your next run and move up your training to the half marathon and beyond is enhanced by scheduling the fun sessions first, with 1-3 of them every week.

STAY INJURY-FREE (A TRAINING JOURNAL HELPS)

When injured runners review their journal, they often find the causes of aches and pains. By following the instructions in this book and journaling, you will reduce your injury risk to almost zero. If you've had injuries before, make a list of past problems and repeated challenges. After reading the injury section of this book, make the needed adjustments. As you eliminate the injury stress, you can eliminate most (or all) of your injuries. We have two successful journals available at *www.JeffGalloway.com*.

AVOIDING OVERUSE OR BURNOUT

All of us get the warning signs of overtraining. Unfortunately, we often ignore these or don't know what they are. Your training journal is a wonderful tool for tracking any possible ache, pain, loss of desire, unusual fatigue that lingers, etc. If you develop an injury, you can review your journal and often find the reasons.

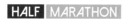

This helps you to become more sensitive to future problems and make conservative adjustments in the plan to reduce upcoming injury risk.

BECOME THE CAPTAIN OF YOUR SHIP

When you balance stress and rest, running bestows a sense of satisfaction and achievement that is unsurpassed. Intuitively, we know that this is good for us, mentally and physically.

When we decide to use the monitoring tools in this book we take a major amount of control over fatigue, injuries, energy level, and enjoyment of running.

WHEN TO SET A TIME GOAL

After finishing your first half marathon you may choose a time goal, after reading the "Choosing the Right Goal" chapter. Many veterans (myself included) decide to stay within current capabilities, use the "to finish" schedule, and enjoy the experience.

I commend all who decide to take on an endurance challenge. Almost everyone who makes it to the finish line will tap into a mysterious and complex source of continuing strength when the elements are balanced. Enjoy the journey!

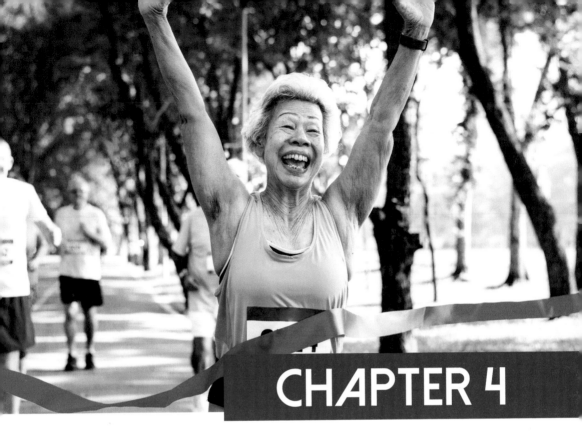

CHAPTER 4

IMPORTANT HEALTH INFORMATION

MEDICAL CHECK

While unlikely that you be advised not to run a half marathon, it's always a good idea to check with your doctor's office before you start a strenuous training program. Keep the doctor informed of cardiovascular system irregularities or aches and pains that could be injuries. At first, just tell your physician or head nurse how much running you plan to be doing over the next year. Almost every person will be given the green light. If your doctor recommends against your running plans, ask why. Since there are so few people who cannot train even for strenuous goals (if they use a liberal Run-Walk-Run formula), I suggest that you get a second opinion if your doctor tells you not to run. Certainly the tiny number of people who should not run have good reasons. But the best medical advisor is one who wants you to get the type of physical activity that engages you – unless there are significant reasons not to do so.

RISKS: HEART DISEASE, LUNG INFECTIONS, SPEEDWORK INJURIES

Running tends to offer an effect that protects against cardiovascular disease. More runners die of heart disease than any other cause and are susceptible to the same risk factors as sedentary people. Like most other people, runners at risk usually don't often realize it.

I know of a number of runners who have suffered heart attacks and strokes who probably could have prevented them if they had taken a few simple tests. Some of these are listed next, but check with your doctor if you have any questions or concerns.

Your heart is the most important organ in your body. This short section is offered as an overview of cardiovascular issues as you maintain a high level of conditioning in the most important organ for longevity and quality of life.

As always, when there are medical issues, you need to get advice about your individual situation from a cardiologist who knows your medical history/condition.

RISK FACTORS – GET CHECKED IF YOU HAVE TWO OF THESE OR ONE THAT IS SERIOUS

- Family history of cardiovascular problems
- Poor lifestyle habits earlier in life (alcohol, drugs, poor diet, etc.)
- High fat/high cholesterol diet
- Have smoked or still smoke
- Obese or severely overweight
- High blood pressure
- High cholesterol
- Diabetes

TESTS

- Stress test – heart is monitored during a run that gradually increases in difficulty

- C-reactive protein – has been an indicator of increased risk

- Radioactive dye test – very effective in locating specific blockages. Talk to your doctor about this.

- Carotid ultrasound test – helps to tell if you're at risk for stroke

- Ankle-brachial test – can detect plaque buildup in arteries throughout the body

None of these tests are foolproof. But by working with your cardiologist, you can increase your chance of living until the muscles just won't propel you farther down the road – maybe beyond the age of 100.

SHOULD I RUN *WHEN* I *HAVE A* COLD?

There are so many individual health issues with a cold that you must talk with a doctor before you exercise when you have an infection.

Lung infection – don't run! A virus in the lungs can move into the heart and kill you. Lung infections are usually indicated by coughing.

Common cold – There are many infections that initially indicate a normal cold but are not – they may be much more serious. At least call your doctor's office to get clearance before running. Be sure to explain how much you are running, and what, if any, medication you are taking.

Infections of the throat and above the neck – most runners will be given the OK, but check with the doctor.

RISK OF SPEED

There is an increased risk of both injuries and cardiovascular events during speed sessions. Be sure to get your doctor's OK before beginning a speed program. The advice inside this book is generally conservative, but when in doubt, take more rest, more days off, and run slower. In other words, be more conservative.

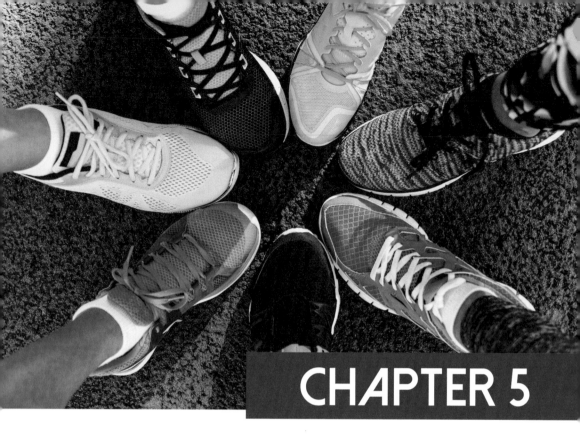

CHAPTER 5

PRACTICAL INFORMATION: SHOES AND EQUIPMENT

One of the wonderful aspects of running, in a complex world, is the simplicity of the experience. You can run from your house or office in most cases, using public streets or pedestrian walkways. Ordinary clothing works well most of the time and you don't need to join a country club or invest in expensive exercise equipment. While running with another person can be motivating, most runners enjoy running alone on most of their runs. It helps, however, to have a "support team" as you go through the training (running companions, doctors, running shoe experts) and you'll probably meet these folks through the running grapevine.

CONVENIENCE

If you have an option near home and office for each of the training components previously listed, you will be more likely to do the workouts on your schedule – when you need to do them.

SHOES

The primary investment: usually less than $118 and more than $79.

After 40 years of observing runners choose shoes in my Atlanta Phidippides stores, I find that most runners decide to spend a little time on the choice of a good running shoe. After all, shoes are the primary equipment needed. The shoe that is a good match for your feet can make running easier, while reducing blisters, foot fatigue, and injuries.

Because there are so many different brands and models, shoe shopping can be confusing. The best advice....is to get the best advice. Going to a good running store, staffed by helpful and knowledgeable runners, can cut the time required and can usually lead you to a much better shoe choice than you would find by yourself. For more information on this, see *Galloway's Book on Running* and the back section of this book.

BUY THE TRAINING SHOE FIRST

Go to the running store in your area with the most experienced staff. First, you'll need a pair for long runs and easy running days. Veterans may want to get a racing shoe (or lightweight training shoe) later. Bring along your most worn pair of shoes (any shoes), and a pair of running shoes that has worked well for you. Wait until you are several weeks into your training before you decide to get a racing shoe if you feel you need one.

DO I NEED A RACING SHOE?

In most cases, racing shoes only speed you up by a few seconds a mile – but this may be what a veteran needs to reach a significant goal. After several weeks, if you feel that your training shoes are too heavy or "clunky," look at some lighter models. After you have broken them in, you can use the lighter shoes during speed sessions.

A WATCH

There are a lot of good, inexpensive watches that will give you accurate times during speed workouts and races. Any watch that has a stopwatch function will do the job. Be sure to ask the staff person in the store how to use the stopwatch function.

A RUN-WALK-RUN TIMER

There is a Galloway timer that can be set for any two intervals desired. It can either "beep" or vibrate or both. For more information or to order this, go to *www.JeffGalloway.com*.

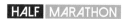

CLOTHING: COMFORT ABOVE ALL

The "clothing thermometer" at the end of this book is a great guide. In the summer, you want to wear light, cool clothing. During cold weather, layering is the best strategy. You don't have to have the latest techno-garments to run. On most days an old pair of shorts and a T-shirt are fine. As you get into the various components of your plan, you will find outfits that make you feel better and motivate you to get in your run even on bad weather days. It is also OK to give yourself a fashionable outfit as a "reward" for running regularly for several weeks.

A TRAINING JOURNAL

The journal is such an important component in running that we have written a chapter about it. By using it to plan ahead and then later, to review your success and mistakes, you assume a major degree of control over your running future. You'll find it reinforcing to write down what you did each day, and miss that reinforcement when you skip. Be sure to read the training journal chapter, and youl too, can steer yourself toward enjoyment and success.

WHERE TO RUN

It helps to have several different venues for the various workouts. Try to find two or more options for each:

Long runs – scenic, interesting areas are best with some pavement and some softer surface if possible. Flatter courses are recommended.

Pace work – a track or any accurately measured segment.

Races and tests – look carefully at the course; avoid hills, too many turns, or even too much flat terrain if you usually train on rolling hills (in a non-hilly race, you will fatigue your flat running muscles more quickly, if you don't run long runs on flat terrain). Read the section on racing.

Drills – any safe running area with a secure surface.

SAFETY – TOP PRIORITY!

Pick a course that is away from car traffic, and is in a safe area – where crime is unlikely. Try to have two or more options for each of the components because variety can be very motivating.

SURFACE

With the correct Run-Walk-Run strategy, adequate amount of cushion, and the right shoes for you, pavement should not give extra shock to the legs or body. A smooth surface dirt or gravel path is best for most runners on the easy days. But beware of uneven surfaces – especially if you have weak ankles or foot problems. For your Magic Miles, speedwork, and drills, you may have to talk to your shoe experts to avoid blisters, etc. when running on certain types of surfaces. Watch the slant of the road, trail, track, or sidewalk – flat is best.

PICKING A RUNNING COMPANION

On long runs and on easy days, don't run with someone who is faster than you unless she is fully comfortable slowing down to an easy pace – that is, slow for you. It is motivating to run with someone who will go slow enough so that you can talk. Share stories, jokes, or even problems if you wish, and you'll bond together in a very positive way. The friendships forged on runs can be the strongest and longest lasting – if you're not huffing and puffing (or puking) from trying to run at a pace that is too fast. On speed days, however, it sometimes helps to run with a faster person as long as you are running at the pace you should be running in each workout.

Note: It is wonderful to run with your husband if the pace is comfortable for both of you. When the pace is too fast for either, the run can be difficult and can lead to injury. As in all such issues, honest discussion is the best policy.

REWARDS

Rewards are important at all times. Be sensitive and provide reinforcements that will keep you motivated and make the running experience a better one (more comfortable shoes, clothes, etc.).

Positive reinforcement works! Treating yourself to a smoothie after a hard run, taking a cool dip in a pool, going out to a special restaurant after a longer run – all of these can reinforce the successful completion of another week or month. Of particular benefit is having a snack, within 30 minutes of the finish of a run, that has 200-300 calories, containing 80% carbohydrate and 20% protein. The products Accelerade and Endurox R4 are already formulated with this ratio for your convenience and give you a recovery boost also.

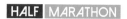

AN APPOINTMENT ON THE CALENDAR OR IN YOUR TRAINING JOURNAL

Write down each of your weekly runs, transposed from the schedule in this book, at least one week in advance, on your calendar or journal. Since each week is broken down for you in this book, you can use it as your guide. Sure, you can change if you have to. But by having a secure running slot, you will be able to plan for your run and make it happen. Pretend that this is an appointment with your boss or your most important client, etc. Actually, you are your most important client!

MOTIVATION TO GET OUT THE DOOR

The three top times when runners feel challenged to run are the following:

1. early in the morning,

2. after work, or

3. before the tough workouts.

In the motivation section, there are rehearsals for challenging situations. You will find it much easier to be motivated once you experience a regular series of runs that make you feel good. When you run and walk at the right pace, with the right preparation, you feel better, can relate to others better, and have more energy to enjoy the rest of the day.

TREADMILLS ARE JUST AS GOOD AS STREETS FOR SHORT RUNS

More and more runners (especially those with small children) are using treadmills for at least 50% of their runs. It is a fact that treadmills tend to tell you that you have gone farther or faster than you really have (but usually are not off by more than 10%). But if you run on a treadmill for the number of minutes assigned, at the effort level you are used to (no huffing and puffing), you will get close enough to the training effect you wish. To ensure that you have run enough miles, feel free to add 10% to your assigned mileage. It's best to run the long runs on the surface used during your goal race.

USUALLY NO NEED TO EAT BEFORE THE RUN

Most runners don't need to eat before runs that are less than 6 miles. The only common exceptions are those with diabetes or severe blood sugar problems. Many runners feel better during a run when they have enjoyed a cup of coffee about 60 minutes before the start. Caffeine engages the central nervous system, which gets all of the systems needed for exercise up and running to capacity very quickly.

If your blood sugar is low, which often occurs in the afternoon, it helps to have a snack of about 100-200 calories, about 30 minutes before the run, that is composed of 80% carbohydrate and 20% protein. The Accelerade product has been in balancing blood sugar levels.

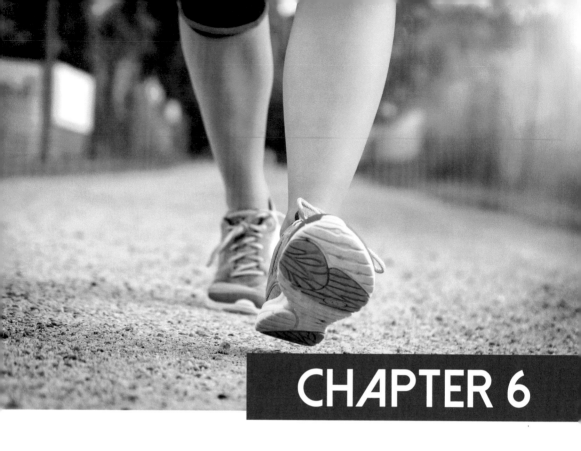

CHAPTER 6

THE GALLOWAY RUN-WALK-RUN METHOD

"Run strong to the end...recover fast...almost eliminate injury...run faster"

The correct Run-Walk-Run strategy in long runs and races can allow you to carry on all of your life activities – even after long runs. The strategy gives you control over your fatigue. Here's how it works.

*WA*LK BEFORE YOU GET TIRED

Most of us, even when untrained, can walk for several miles before fatigue sets in because walking is an activity that we can do efficiently for hours. Running is more work because you have to lift your body off the ground and then absorb the shock of the landing, over and over. The continuous use of the running muscles will produce much more fatigue, aches, and pains than maintaining the same pace while taking walk breaks. If you walk before your running muscles start to get tired, you allow the muscle to recover instantly, increasing your capacity for exercise while reducing the chance of next-day soreness.

The "method" part involves having a strategy. By using a ratio of running and walking that is right for you on each day, you can manage your fatigue. You are the one who is strong to the finish, doing what you need or want to do after long runs. You never have to be exhausted after a long run again.

"The run-walk method is very simple: you run for a short segment and then take a walk break, and keep repeating this pattern."

WALK BREAKS ...

- Speed you up: An average of 7 minutes faster in a 13.1 when non-stop runners shift to the correct Run-Walk-Run ratio
- Give you control over the way you feel at the end
- Ease fatigue
- Push back your fatigue wall
- Allow for endorphins to collect during each walk break – you feel good!
- Break up the distance into manageable units ("two more minutes")
- Speed recovery
- Reduce the chance of aches, pains, and injury
- Allow you to feel good afterward – carrying on the rest of your day without debilitating fatigue
- Give you all of the endurance of the distance of each session without the pain
- Allow older runners or heavier runners to recover fast and feel as good or better as the younger (slimmer) days
- Activate the frontal lobe – keeping you in control over your attitude and motivation

A SHORT AND GENTLE WALKING STRIDE

It's better to walk slowly with a short stride. There has been some irritation of the shins when runners or walkers maintain a stride that is too long. Relax and enjoy the walk.

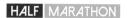

NO NEED TO ELIMINATE THE WALK BREAKS

Some beginners assume that they must work toward the day when they don't have to take any walk breaks at all. This is up to the individual but is not recommended. Remember that you decide what ratio of Run-Walk-Run to use. There is no rule that requires you to hold to any ratio on a given day. As you adjust the run-walk to how you feel, you gain control over your fatigue.

I've run for over 60 years, and I enjoy running more than ever because of walk breaks. Each run I take energizes my day. I would not be able to run almost every day if I didn't insert the walk breaks early and often.

HOW TO KEEP TRACK OF THE WALK BREAKS

The best product is the Galloway Run-Walk-Run timer, which will beep or vibrate. There are several watches that can be set for two intervals. Check our website *(www.jeffgalloway. com)*.

RUN-WALK-RUN RATIOS

After having heard back from over 500,000 runners who have used walk breaks at various paces, I've come up with the following suggested ratios:

Pace/mile	Run	Walk
7:00	6 min	30 sec (or run one mile/walk 40 seconds)
7:30	5 min	30 sec (or 2:30/15)
8:00	4 min	30 sec (or 2/15)
8:30	3 min	30 sec (or 2/23)
9:00	2 min	30 sec or 80/20
9:30 -10:45	R90sec/W30sec or R60sec/W20sec or R45sec/W15sec or R60sec/W30sec or R40sec/W20sec	
10:45-12:15	R60sec/W30sec or R40sec/W20sec or R30sec/W15sec or R30sec/W30sec or R20sec/W20sec	
12:15-14:30	R30sec/W30sec or R20sec/W20sec or R15sec/W15sec	
14:30-15:45	R15sec/W30sec	
15:45-17:00	R10sec/W30sec	
17:00-18:30	R8sec/W30sec or R5sec/W25sec or R10sec/W30sec	
18:30-20:00	R5sec/W30sec or R5sec/W25sec or R4sec/W30sec	

R3min/W30sec = Run 3 minutes/Walk 30 seconds

Note: You may always divide each of the amounts by 2. Example: instead of running 9min/mi pace using 4-1, you could run for 2 minutes and walk for 30 seconds.

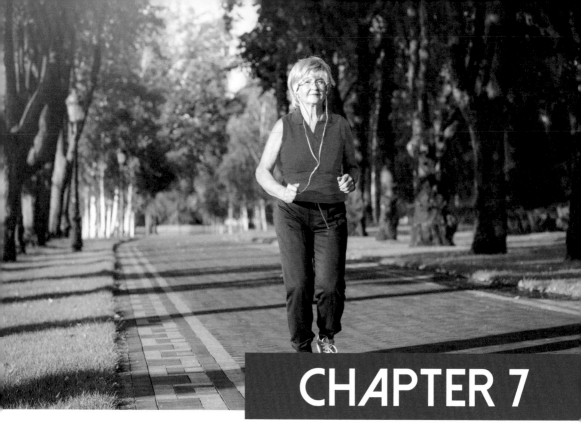

CHAPTER 7

CHOOSING THE RIGHT GOAL AND PACE

In this chapter, you'll learn how to determine the right pace for your long runs and the race itself. Veterans will learn how much improvement can be expected and whether they are on track for their goals at various times in the training program. As you approach your goal at the end of the program, you can use the "Galloway Performance Predictor" to determine what you will be capable of running in your race and how to make adjustments for temperature.

PREDICTION STRATEGY

Several decades ago, I started using a one-mile time trial (called the "Magic Mile") as a prediction tool. After working with hundreds and then thousands of runners, I've found that those who do 3-4 of these during a season can accurately predict their current half marathon racing potential. By adding 3 min/mi to this time, runners will find an injury-reducing pace for the long runs.

In order to run the time in the race indicated by Galloway's Performance Predictor:

- You have done the training necessary for the goal – according to the training programs in this book

- You are not injured

- You run with an even-paced effort

- The weather on goal race day is not adverse (race day temps are below 60F or 14C, no strong headwinds, no heavy rain or snow, etc.)

- There are no crowds to run through or significant hills

THE "MAGIC MILE" TIME TRIAL (MM)

- These time trials are listed on the schedules in this book.

- Go to a track, or other accurately measured course. One mile is 4 laps around a standard track (400 meters).

- Warm up by walking for 5 minutes, then by using a Run-Walk-Run strategy that is more conservative than you will use in your "Magic Mile." If you plan to use a 3 min run/30 sec walk later in the run then as you warm up, run a minute and walk for 20-30 seconds. Then, for 5-10 minutes, jog at an easy pace, with walk breaks as desired.

- Do 4 acceleration gliders. These are listed in the "Drills" chapter.

- Walk for 3-4 minutes.

- Run fast – for you – for 4 laps. Use walk break suggestions in this chapter or run the way you want – never sprint.

- On your first MM, don't run all-out from the start – just run a normal pace for 3 laps and pick it up a little. Be sure to record your time.

- Cool down by reversing the warm-up.

- A school track is the best venue. Don't use a treadmill because they tend to be notoriously uncalibrated and often tell you that you ran farther or faster than you really did.

- On each successive MM, try to adjust pace in order to run a faster time.

- Use the following formula to see what time is predicted in the goal races.

HOW HARD SHOULD I RUN THE MM?

The first one should be only slightly faster than you normally run. With each successive MM, pick up the pace and try to beat your previous best time. By the fourth MM, you should be running fairly close to your potential.

Run the first lap slightly slower than you think you can average. Take a short walk break as noted in the walk break suggestions in this chapter. If you aren't huffing and puffing you can pick up the pace a bit on the second lap. If you are huffing after the first lap, then just hold your pace on lap two – or reduce it slightly. Most runners benefit from taking a walk break after the second lap. At the end of lap 3, the walk break is optional. It is OK to be breathing hard on the last lap. If you are slowing down on the last lap, start a little slower on the next MM. When you finish, you should feel like you couldn't run more than about half a lap at that pace. You may find that you don't need many (or any) walk breaks during the MM – experiment and adjust.

GALLOWAY'S PERFORMANCE PREDICTOR

STEP 1:

Run your "Magic Mile" time trial (MM) (4 laps around the track).

STEP 2:

Convert minutes and seconds to minutes and 1/100ths. Example: 9:30 is 9.5.

MM Time	(x 1.2) FAST Half Mar Pace	(add 3 min/mi) Long Run Training Pace
5:00	6:00	9:00
5:30	6:37	9:40
6:00	7:12	10:15
6:30	7:48	10:50
7:00	8:24	11:30
7:30	9:00	12:00
8:00	9:36	12:40
8:30	10:12	13:15
9:00	10:48	13:50
9:30	11:24	14:30
10:00	12:00	15:00
10:30	12:36	15:40
11:00	13:12	16:15
11:30	13:48	16:50
12:00	14:24	17:30
12:30	15:00	18:00
13:00	15:36	18:40
13:30	16:12	19:15
14:00	16:48	19:50
14:30	17:24	20:30
15:00	18:00	21:00
15:30	18:36	21:40
16:00	19:12	22:15

Note: The 1.2 multiplier assumes that you will be running about all-out effort by the end of the half marathon.

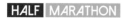

FIRST-TIME HALF MARATHONERS - RUN TO FINISH ONLY

I strongly recommend that first-time half marathon runners should not attempt a time goal. Use the "Magic Mile" to determine your long run pace (adding 3 minutes to the time multiplied by 1.2). During the race itself, I recommend running the first 10 miles at your training pace. During the last 3 miles, you may run as you wish.

TIME GOAL RUNNERS
MAY MAKE A "LEAP OF FAITH" GOAL PREDICTION

I have no problem allowing my e-coach athletes, who've run one or more half marathons, to choose a goal time that is faster than that predicted by the initial MM. As you do the speed training, the long runs and your test races, you should improve – but how much? In my experience, this "leap of faith" should not exceed 3-5% improvement in a 3-month training program.

- Run the MM

- Use the formula above to predict what you could run now, if you were trained for the half marathon

- Choose the amount of improvement during the training program (3-5%)

HOW MUCH OF A "LEAP OF FAITH" IMPROVEMENT?

Half-marathon pre-test prediction	* 3% Improvement	* 5% Improvement
	(Over a 2-3 month training program)	
1:20	2:12	4:00
1:40	3:00	5:00
2:00	3:36	6:00
2:30	4:30	7:30
3:00	5:24	9:00

Finish time improvement half marathon pre-test prediction	3%	5%
3:00	2:54:36	2:51:00
2:30	2:25:30	2:22:30
2:00	1:56:24	1:54:00

The key to goal setting is keeping your ego in check. From my experience, I have found that a 3% improvement is realistic. This means that if your half marathon time is predicted to be 3:00, then it is realistic to assume you could lower it by five and a half minutes if you do the speed training and the long runs as noted on my training schedules in this book. The maximum improvement, which is less likely, is a more aggressive 5% or 9 minutes off a three-hour half marathon.

In both of these situations, however, everything must come together to produce the predicted result. Even runners who shoot for a 3% improvement do all the training as described and achieve their goal slightly more than 50% of the time during a racing season. The more aggressive performances usually result in success about 20% of the time. There are many factors that determine a time goal in a half marathon that are outside of your control: weather, terrain, infection, etc.

The prediction from the MM assumes that you have done all of the training for the goal (long runs and speed workouts) in this book, weather is ideal, the course is not hilly, and there is not a lot of weaving runners ahead – or swinging wide around turns.

"MAGIC MILE" TIME TRIALS (MM) GIVE YOU A REALITY CHECK

- Follow the same format as listed in the pre-test.
- By doing this as noted, you will learn how to pace yourself.
- Hint: it's better to start a bit more slowly than you think you can run.
- Walk breaks will be helpful for most runners. Read the section in this book for suggested ratios.
- Note whether you are speeding up or slowing down at the end, and adjust in the next MM.
- If you are not making progress then look for reasons and take action.

REASONS WHY YOU MAY NOT BE IMPROVING:

- You're overtrained, and tired – if so, reduce your training, and take an extra rest day.

- You may have chosen a goal that is too ambitious for your current ability.

- You may have missed some of your workouts or not been as regular with your training as needed.

- The temperature may have been above 60F (14C). Above this, you will slow down (the longer the race, the more slowdown due to heat).

- You ran the first lap or two too fast.

FINAL REALITY CHECK

Time goal runners: Take your fastest MM and multiply by 1.2. It is recommended that you run the first third of your goal race a few seconds per mile slower than the pace predicted by the MM.

"To finish" runners should run the first 8-10 miles at training pace and then speed up if desired.

If the MMs are predicting a time that is slower than the goal you've been training for, go with the time predicted by the "Magic Mile."

USE A JOURNAL!

Read the chapter on using a journal. Your chance of achieving your goal increases greatly with this very important instrument. Psychologically, you start taking responsibility for the fulfillment of your mission when you use a journal.

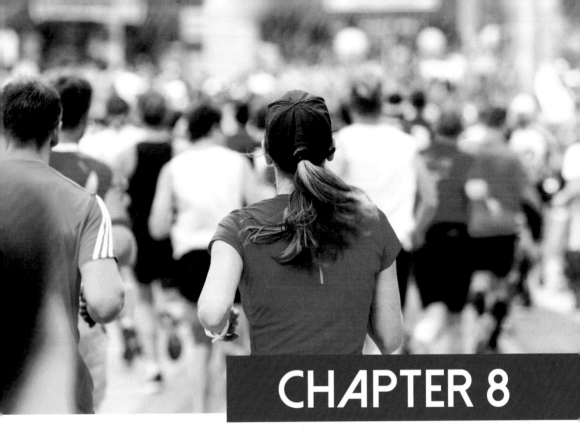

CHAPTER 8

PRIMARY TRAINING COMPONENTS

LONG RUNS

Run these very slowly, at least 3 min/mi slower than you could run in a half marathon as predicted by your MM. Insert the walk breaks as suggested in the Run-Walk-Run chapter in this book – or more often. I have not found anyone who has run the long runs too slowly or has taken the walk breaks too often. Slower long runs build the same endurance as fast long runs – with reduced risk of injury or burnout.

DRILLS

Cadence Drills (CD) and Acceleration Gliders (AG). These easy exercises teach your body to improve form, as you improve running mechanics. They are not exhausting; most runners say they energize an average run. Doing each of these drills once a week can improve speed and running efficiency.

HILLS

Hills build running strength better than any other training component. Warm up by jogging slowly for a half mile. Then, do 4 acceleration gliders (AG). Start each hill at a jog, and pick up the turnover as you go over the top of the hill. Don't sprint, but you will be huffing and puffing. Shorten stride slightly as you go up the hill. See the section in this book on hill training.

"MAGIC MILE" TIME TRIALS (MM)

These are done every few weeks to monitor progress and overtraining.

- Go to a track, or other accurately measured course.

- Warm up by walking for 5 minutes, then running a minute and walking a minute, then jogging an easy 800 meters (half mile or two laps around a track).

- Do 4 acceleration gliders. These are listed in the "Drills" chapter.

- Walk for 3-4 minutes.

- Run the 1 mile MM – a hard effort. Follow the walk break suggestions.

- On your first MM, don't run all-out from the start – ease into your pace after the first third of the distance.

- Cool down by reversing the warm-up.

- A school track is the best venue. Don't use a treadmill because they tend to be notoriously uncalibrated and often tell you that you ran farther or faster than you really did. Run the first lap slightly slower than you think you can average. Take a short walk break as noted in the walk break suggestions in this chapter. It is OK to be huffing and puffing on the last lap. If you are slowing down on the last lap, start a little slower on the next one. When you finish, you should feel like you couldn't run more than about half a lap further at that pace.

FOR TIME-GOAL RUNNERS

Speed(s) – A gradual increase in speed training can prepare you for the realistic goal of your choice. See the speedwork section of this book.

Pace(p) – On these runs, you want to run at race pace, taking various Run-Walk-Run strategies you might use in the race. This is like a dress rehearsal for race day. By finding the right strategy and practicing at race pace, you will be ready.

- Warm up with 5 min of walking, then 10 min of easy running and walking.
- Time yourself for a segment that is between half a mile and 1 mile.
- Run at your goal pace.
- Insert various Run-Walk-Run strategies to see what works best for you.
- Do 1-2 miles of these segments.
- Don't do them if your legs are too tired.
- Reverse the warm-up as a cool-down.

TRACK DISTANCES

400 meters is approximately a quarter of a mile or one lap around a track; 1 mi is one mile, or 4 laps around a track

These diverse elements are woven together throughout the training season so that you can continue to improve speed and endurance. The whole process is like a symphony of elements that blend mind and body, heart, and legs, left brain and right into an integrated unit.

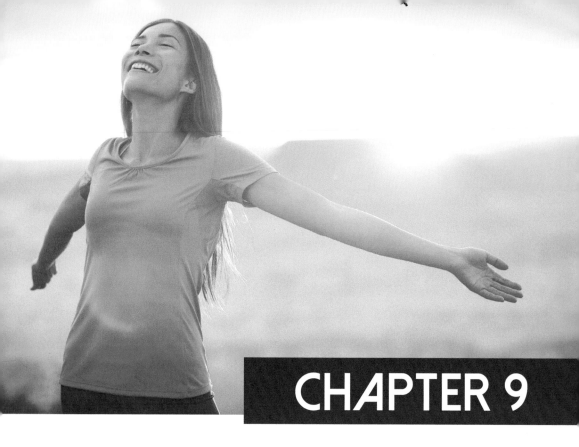

CHAPTER 9

BODY, MIND, AND SPIRIT RESPOND POSITIVELY TO TRAINING

THE "TEAM" OF HEART, LUNGS, NERVES, BRAIN, ETC.

Very often in college and professional sports, a group of very talented individuals is defeated by players of lesser ability who play as a team. In a similar way, running helps to mold your key body components into a coordinated unit. When running within one's capacity, the left side of the frontal lobe sets up a cognitive plan and the right side uses its intuitive and creative powers to solve problems, manage resources, and help us find the pace and amount of training that we can handle. While the heart is our primary blood pump, leg muscles, when fit, will provide significant help in pushing blood back to the heart.

THE HEART GETS STRONGER

Like any muscle, the heart's strength and effectiveness is increased through regular endurance exercise.

THE LUNGS

The lungs become more efficient in processing oxygen and inserting it into the blood.

ENDORPHINS

Endorphins (natural painkillers) reduce discomfort and give you a relaxing and positive attitude.

THE LONG RUN BUILDS ENDURANCE

By gradually extending slow long runs, you train muscle cells to expand their capacity to utilize oxygen efficiently, sustain energy production, and, in general, increase capacity to go farther. The continued increase in the distance of these long runs increases the reach of blood artery capillaries to deliver oxygen and improves the return of waste products so that the muscles can work at top capacity. In short, long runs bestow a better plumbing system, improving muscle capacity. These changes will pay off at the end of your half marathon.

Even when running very slowly, with liberal walk breaks, you build endurance by gradually increasing the distance of a regularly scheduled long run. Start with the length of your current long one and increase as noted in the following schedule.

MAINTAIN CURRENT ENDURANCE

With two 30-minute runs, every other day (e.g., Tuesday and Thursday).

A half-hour run on Tuesday and Thursday will maintain the endurance gained on the weekend. This is the minimum and results in the lowest injury rate. If you are already running more than this, without aches and pains, you can continue if you wish – but be careful.

To summarize, the long runs on weekends, with two other runs during the week, will create a level of fitness and muscle strength sufficient to prepare for your goal in the half marathon. At the same time, you'll be improving the internal engineering of the muscles: enhanced oxygen absorption, increased blood flow, better energy supply and storage, and much more. Hills, speedwork, and form drills improve the mechanical efficiency of the bones, muscles, and tendons as they adapt, helping you to become a more efficient runner.

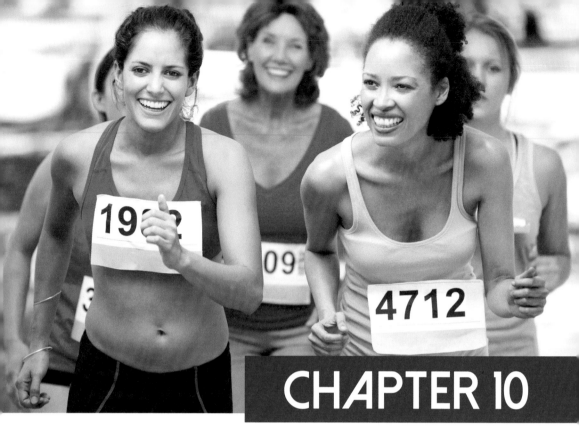

CHAPTER 10

HALF MARATHON TRAINING PROGRAMS

BEGINNER

To find per kilometer pace, convert mile pace to a decimal and multiply by .62. For example, 10:24 per mile would be 10.4 x .62 = 6.448 which = 6:27/km.

1. This program is designed for those who have not been running regularly for a month or more. If you are already running more than 1 mile, you can begin on the week corresponding to your longest run in the last two weeks.

2. What pace should you run on the long runs? Read the chapter in this book on "Choosing the Right Goal." After you run the one-mile MM (time trial), multiply by 1.2, then add 3 minutes – the result is your pace-per-mile on long runs at 60F (14C) or cooler.

3. Run-Walk-Run ratio should correspond to the pace used, as noted in the Run-Walk-Run chapter of this book.

4. Pace for the half marathon itself: Run the first 10 miles at the training pace noted. If you want speed up a little, you can do so during the last 3 miles.

5. On long runs and the race itself, slow down when the temperature rises above 60F (14C) by 30 sec a mile for every 5 degrees above 60F or more (or by 20 sec/ kilometer for every 2 degrees of temperature increase above 14C).

6. Tuesday and Thursday runs can be done at the pace of your choice.

7. It is fine to do cross-training on Monday, Wednesday, and Friday, if you wish. There will be little benefit to your running in doing this, but you'll increase your fat-burning capacity. On these recovery days, don't do exercises like stair machines that use the calf muscles.

8. Be sure to take a vacation from strenuous exercise the day before your weekend runs.

Mon	Tue	Wed	Thu	Fri	Sat	Sun
1. off	30 min run	off	30 min run	easy walk	off	1 mile
2. off	30 min run	off	30 min run(TT)	easy walk	off	1.5 miles
3. off	30 min run	off	30 min run(TT)	easy walk	off	2.0 miles
4. off	30 min run	off	30 min run(TT)	easy walk	off	2.5 miles
5. off	30 min run	off	30 min run(TT)	easy walk	off	3 miles
6. off	30 min run	off	30 min run	easy walk	off	2.0 miles
7. off	30 min run	off	30 min run	easy walk	off	4.0 miles
8. off	30 min run	off	30 min run	easy walk	off	5K event
9. off	30 min run	off	30 min run	easy walk	off	5.0 miles
10. off	30 min run	off	30 min run	easy walk	off	2.5 miles
11. off	30 min run	off	30 min run	easy walk	off	6.0 miles TT + 2 mi
12. off	30 min run	off	30 min run	easy walk	off	3.0 miles
13. off	30 min run	off	30 min run	easy walk	off	7.0 miles
14. off	30 min run	off	30 min run	easy walk	off	3.0 miles
15. off	30 min run	off	30 min run	easy walk	off	8.0 miles
16. off	30 min run	off	30 min run	easy walk	off	3.0 miles

Mon	Tue	Wed	Thu	Fri	Sat	Sun
17. off	30 min run	off	30 min run	easy walk	off	9.0 miles
18. off	30 min run	off	30 min run	easy walk	off	3.0 miles with MM
19. off	30 min run	off	30 min run	easy walk	off	10 miles
20. off	30 min run	off	30 min run	easy walk	off	3.0 miles with MM
21. off	30 min run	off	30 min run	easy walk	off	11 miles
22. off	30 min run	off	30 min run	easy walk	off	3 mi with MM
23. off	30 min run	off	30 min run	easy walk	off	12 miles
24. off	30 min run	off	30 min run	easy walk	off	3 mi with MM
25. off	30 min run	off	30 min run	easy walk	off	13 miles
26. off	30 min run	off	30 min run	easy walk	off	3 mi with MM
27. off	30 min run	off	30 min run	easy walk	off	14 miles
28. off	30 min run	off	30 min run	easy walk	off	3 mi
29. off	30 min run	off	30 min run	easy walk	off	HMR*
30. off	30 min run	off	30 min run	easy walk	off	3.0 miles
31. off	30 min run	off	30 min run	easy walk	off	13 miles
32. off	30 min run	off	30 min run	easy walk	off	1 mi TT + 3 mi
33. off	30 min run	off	30 min run	easy walk	off	14 miles
34. off	30 min run	off	30 min run	easy walk	off	4.0 miles
35. off	30 min run	off	30 min run	easy walk	off	Half marathon!
36. off	30 min run	off	30 min run	easy walk	off	3-4 miles
37. off	30 min run	off	30 min run	easy walk	off	5-6 miles
38. off	30 min run	off	30 min run	easy walk	off	5-13 miles

* HMR: Half Marathon Race

TO FINISH

To find per kilometer pace, convert mile pace to a decimal and multiply by .62. For example, 10:24 per mile would be 10.4 x .62 = 6.448 which = 6:27/km.

1. This program is designed for those who have already been running regularly, but have never run a half marathon before, or for veterans who don't have a time goal. To begin this program, you should have a long run within the past two weeks of at least 7 miles. If your long run is not this long, then gradually increase the weekend run to this distance before beginning this program.

2. What pace should you run on the long runs? Read the chapter in this book on "Choosing the Right Goal." After you run the first MM ("Magic Mile"), multiply by 1.2, then add 3 minutes – the result is your suggested long run pace per mile on long runs at 60F (14C) or cooler.

3. Run-Walk-Run ratio should correspond to the pace used.

4. Pace for the half marathon itself: Run the first 9 miles at the training pace noted. If you want to speed up a little, you can do so at that point.

5. On long runs and the race itself, slow down when the temperature rises above 60F (14C) by 30 sec a mile for every 5 degrees above 60F or more (20 sec/km slower for every 2C above 14C).

6. Tuesday and Thursday runs can be done at the pace of your choice.

7. It is fine to do cross-training on Monday, Wednesday, and Friday if you wish. There will be little benefit to your running in doing this, but you'll increase your fat burning. Don't do exercises like stair machines that use the calf muscle.

8. Be sure to take a vacation from strenuous exercise the day before your weekend runs.

9. An optional pace mile (p) is noted on the Thursday run. To get used to a pace you want to run at the end of the half marathon, time yourself for a mile and take the walk breaks as you will do them in the race.

Mon	Tue	Wed	Thu	Fri	Sat	Sun
1. off	30 min run	off	30 min run(MM)	easy walk	off	8 miles
2. off	30 min run	off	30 min run	easy walk	off	1 mi MM + 3 mi
3. off	30 min run	off	30 min run(MM)	easy walk	off	9 miles
4. off	30 min run	off	30 min run(MM)	easy walk	off	4 miles
5. off	30 min run	off	30 min run	easy walk	off	10 miles
6. off	30 min run	off	30 min run	easy walk	off	1 mi MM + 4 mi
7. off	30 min run	off	30 min run	easy walk	off	11 miles
8. off	30 min run	off	30 min run	easy walk	off	5 miles
9. off	30 min run	off	30 min run	easy walk	off	12 miles
10. off	30 min run	off	30 min run	easy walk	off	1 mi MM + 4 mi
11. off	30 min run	off	30 min run	easy walk	off	13 miles
12. off	30 min run	off	30 min run	easy walk	off	5 miles
13. off	30 min run	off	30 min run	easy walk	off	14 miles
14. off	30 min run	off	30 min run	easy walk	off	1 mi MM + 4 mi
15. off	30 min run	off	30 min run	easy walk	off	Half marathon
16. off	30 min run	off	30 min run	easy walk	off	3-5 miles

TIME GOAL PROGRAM: 2:30-3:00

To find per kilometer pace, convert mile pace to a decimal and multiply by .62. For example, 10:24 per mile would be 10.4 x .62 = 6.448 which = 6:27/km.

> **Note:** This is the minimum that I've found necessary to prepare for the goal. If you are already running more than this amount and are able to recover between workouts, you may continue what you are doing, but be careful.

1. To begin this program, you should have run a long run within the past two weeks of at least 7 miles. If your long run is not this long, then gradually increase the weekend run to this distance before starting this program.

2. What is my current level of performance? Read the chapter in this book on "Choosing the Right Goal." After you run the first "Magic Mile" (MM), multiply by 1.2. This tells you what you are currently capable of running in a half marathon (per mile) right now when the temperature is 60F (14C) or below, assuming that you have done the long runs and speed training listed in the schedule. If you want to improve, see the "Predicting Race Performance" section in this book.

3. What pace should I run on the long runs? Take your current performance level (one mile MM x 1.2) and add 3 minutes – the result is your suggested long run pace per mile on long runs at 60F (14C) or cooler.

4. On long runs and the race itself, slow down when the temperature rises above 60F (14C) by 30 sec a mile for every 5 degrees above 60F or more (20 sec/km slower for every 2C above 14C).

5. Run-Walk-Run ratio should correspond to the pace used.

6. At the beginning of the program, after you have run the first MM, you can choose a goal that is as fast as 20 seconds per mile (15 sec/km) faster than predicted by the process indicated in number 2 in this section or any goal slower than this. To use this schedule, the goal pace should be between 11:30 and 13:30.

7. To compute your pace for the 800-meter (2 laps around a track) repeats done on speedwork weekends, take half the time of your goal pace per mile, as you decided according to number 6, and subtract 15 seconds. Example: for a 12 min/mi pace, run each 800 in 5:45.

8. Warm up for each 800-meter repeat workout by walking for 5 minutes, then jogging very slowly for 5-10 minutes. Then do 4-8 acceleration gliders (see the segment on drills in this book). Cool down at the end by jogging slowly for 5 minutes and then walking for 5 minutes. Walk 3 min between each 800-meter repeat. At the end of the first lap, walk for 20-30 seconds – but don't stop your stopwatch. The time for each 800 should be from the start until the end of the second lap.

9. If you have recovered from the weekend workout on Tuesday, run some 800s at race pace (noted as "rr" on these particular Tuesdays). After an easy warm-up, run 4 of the cadence drills (CD) and 4 acceleration gliders (AG). These are described in the drill section of this book. Then run 3-4 x half mile (800 meter) segments at goal pace, taking the walk breaks as you plan to do them in the race. Jog for the rest of your run. As the weeks pass, try various ratios of running to walking to see which feels best, running your goal pace.

10. It is fine to do cross-training on Monday, Wednesday, and Friday, if you wish. There will be little benefit to your running in doing this, but you'll increase your fat-burning potential. Don't do exercises like stair machines that use the calf muscle on these recovery days.

11. Be sure to take a vacation from strenuous exercise the day before your weekend runs.

12. On Thursday, run a few hill repeats (h) as described in the hill section in this book – except for the days set aside for the MMs.

Mon	Tue	Wed	Thu	Fri	Sat	Sun
1. off	30 min run	off	30 min run (MM)	easy walk	off	8 miles
2. off	30 min run	off	1 mi MM +1mi	easy walk	off	2 x 800m
3. off	30 min run	off	30 min run (MM)	easy walk	off	9 miles
4. off	30 min run	off	30 min run (MM)	easy walk	off	3 x 800m
5. off	30 min run	off	30 min run	easy walk	off	10 miles
6. off	30 min run	off	1 mi MM 1mi	easy walk	off	4 x 800m
7. off	30 min run	off	30 min run	easy walk	off	11 miles
8. off	30 min run	off	30 min run	easy walk	off	6 x 800m
9. off	30 min run	off	30 min run	easy walk	off	12 miles
10. off	30 min run	off	1 mi MM +1mi	easy walk	off	8 x 800m

Mon	Tue	Wed	Thu	Fri	Sat	Sun
11. off	30 min run	off	30 min run	easy walk	off	13.5 miles
12. off	30 min run	off	30 min run	easy walk	off	10 x 800m
13. off	30 min run	off	30 min run	easy walk	off	15 miles
14. off	30 min run	off	30 min run	easy walk	off	1 mi MM + 3 mi
15. off	30 min run	off	30 min run	easy walk	off	Half marathon
16. off	30 min run	off	30 min run	easy walk	off	3-5 miles

TIME GOAL PROGRAM: 1:59-2:29

To find per kilometer pace, convert mile pace to a decimal and multiply by .62. For example, 10:24 per mile would be 10.4 x .62 = 6.448 which = 6:27/km.

Note: This is the minimum that I've found necessary to prepare for this goal. If you are already running more than this amount, and are able to recover between workouts, you may continue to do what you are doing, but be careful.

1. To begin this program, you should have run a long run within the past two weeks of at least 7 miles. If your long run is not this long, then gradually increase the weekend run to this distance before starting this program.

2. What is my current level of performance? Read the chapter in this book on "Choosing the Right Goal." After you run the first "Magic Mile" (MM), multiply by 1.2. This predicts what you what you are currently capable of running in a half marathon (per mile) right now, when the temperature is 60F or below, and if you have done the long runs and speed training listed in the schedule. If you want to improve, see the "Predicting Race Performance" section in this book.

3. What pace should I run on the long runs? Take your current performance level (MM x 1.2) and add 3 minutes; the result is your suggested long run pace per mile on long runs at 60F (14C) or cooler.

4. On long runs and the race itself, slow down when the temperature rises above 60F (14C) by 30 sec per mile for every 5 degrees above 60F or more. (20 sec/km slower for every 2C above 14C).

5.   Run-Walk-Run ratio should correspond to the pace used.

6.   At the beginning of the program, after you have run the first MM, you can choose a goal that is as fast as 20 seconds per mile (15 sec/km) faster than predicted by the process indicated in number 2 in this section or any goal slower than this. To use this schedule, the goal pace should be between 9:10 and 11:30.

7.   To compute your pace for the 800-meter (2 laps around a track) repeats done on speedwork weekends, take half the time of your goal pace per mile, as you decided according to number 6, and subtract 15 seconds. Example: for a 10 min/mi pace, run each 800 in 4:45. Warm up for each 800-meter repeat workout by walking for 5 minutes, then jogging very slowly for 5-10 minutes. Then do 4-8 acceleration gliders (see the segment on drills in this book). Cool down at the end by jogging slowly for 5 minutes and then walking for 5 minutes. Walk 3 min between each 800-meter repeat. At the end of the first lap, walk for 20-30 seconds – but don't stop your stopwatch. The time for each 800 should be from the start until the end of the second lap.

8.   If you have recovered from the weekend workout on Tuesday, run two "race rehearsal" miles (noted as "rr" on the Tue line). After an easy warm-up, run 4 of the cadence drills (CD) and 4 acceleration gliders (AG). These are described in the drill section of this book. Then run 2-4 x one mile (1600 meter) segments, taking the walk breaks as you plan to do them in the race. Jog for the rest of your run. As the weeks pass, try various ratios of running/walking to see which feels best when running your goal pace.

9.   It is fine to do cross-training on Monday, Wednesday, and Friday, if you wish. There will be little benefit to your running in doing this, but you'll increase your fat-burning potential. Don't do exercises like stair machines that use the calf muscle on these recovery days.

10.   Be sure to take a vacation from strenuous exercise the day before your weekend runs.

11.   On Thursday, run a few hill repeats (h) as described in the hill section in this book – except for the days set aside for the MMs.

Mon	Tue	Wed	Thu	Fri	Sat	Sun
1. off	30-45 min run	off	30-45min (TT)	easy walk	off	8 miles
2. off	30-45 min run	off	1 mi TT +1mi	easy walk	off	3 x 800m
3. off	30-45 min run	off	30-45min(TT)	easy walk	off	9.5 miles
4. off	30-45 min run	off	30-45min(TT)	easy walk	off	5 x 800m
5. off	30-45 min run	off	30-45 min run	easy walk	off	11 miles
6. off	30-45 min run	off	1 mi TT 2mi	easy walk	off	7 x 800m
7. off	30-45 min run	off	30-45 min run	easy walk	off	12.5 miles
8. off	30-45 min run	off	30-45 min run	easy walk	off	9 x 800m
9. off	30-45 min run	off	30-45 min run	easy walk	off	14 miles
10. off	30-45 min run	off	1 mi TT +2mi	easy walk	off	11 x 800m
11. off	30-45 min run	off	30-45 min run	easy walk	off	15 miles
12. off	30-45 min run	off	30-45 min run	easy walk	off	12 x 800m
13. off	30-45 min run	off	30-45 min run	easy walk	off	17 miles
14. off	30-45 min run	off	30-45 min run	easy walk	off	13 x 800m
15. off	30-45 min run	off	30-45 min run	easy walk	off	4 miles
16. off	30-45 min run	off	30-45 min run	easy walk	off	HM*
17. off	30-45 min run	off	30-45 min run	easy walk	off	5 miles

* HM = Half marathon

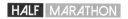

TIME GOAL PROGRAM: 1:45-1:58

To find per kilometer pace, convert mile pace to a decimal and multiply by .62. For example, 10:24 per mile would be 10.4 x .62 = 6.448 which = 6:27/km.

> **Note:** This is the minimum that I've found necessary to prepare for this goal. If you are already running more than this amount, and are able to recover between workouts, you may continue to do what you are doing, but be careful.

1. To begin this program, you should have run a long run within the past two weeks of at least 7 miles. If your long run is not this long, then gradually increase the weekend run to this distance before starting this program.

2. What is my current level of performance? Read the chapter in this book on "Choosing the Right Goal." After you run the first "Magic Mile" (MM), multiply by 1.2. This predicts what you what you are currently capable of running in a half marathon (per mile) right now, when the temperature is 60F or below, and if you have done the long runs and speed training listed in the schedule. If you want to improve, see the "Predicting Race Performance" section in this book.

3. What pace should I run on the long runs? Take your current performance level (MM x 1.2) and add 3 minutes – the result is your suggested long run pace per mile on long runs at 60F(14C) or cooler.

4. On long runs and the race itself, slow down when the temperature rises above 60F (14C) by 30 sec a mile for every 5 degrees above 60F or more (20 sec/km slower for every 2C above 14C).

5. Run-Walk-Run ratio should correspond to the pace used.

6. At the beginning of the program, after you have run the first MM, you can choose a goal that is as fast as 20 seconds per mile (15 sec/km) faster than predicted by the process indicated in number 2 in this section or any goal slower than this. To use this schedule, the goal pace should be between 8:00 and 9:10 per mile.

7. To compute your pace for the 800-meter (2 laps around a track) repeats done on speedwork weekends, take half the time of your goal pace per mile, as you decided according to number 6, and subtract 15 seconds. Example: for a 9 min/mi pace, run each 800 in 4:15.

Mon	Tue	Wed	Thu	Fri	Sat	Sun
1. off	40-60 min run	off	40-60min (MM)	25 min	off	8 miles
2. off	40-60 min run	off	1 mi TT +3mi	25 min	off	5 x 800m
3. off	40-60 min run	off	40-60min (MM)	25 min	off	9.5 miles
4. off	40-60 min run	off	40-60min (MM)	25 min	off	7 x 800m
5. off	40-60 min run	off	40-60 min run	25 min	off	11 miles
6. off	40-60 min run	off	1 mi TT +4mi	25 min	off	9 x 800m
7. off	40-60 min run	off	40-60 min run	25 min	off	12.5 miles
8. off	40-60 min run	off	40-60 min run	25 min	off	11 x 800m
9. off	40-60 min run	off	40-60 min run	25 min	off	14 miles
10. off	40-60 min run	off	1 mi TT +4mi	25 min	off	12 x 800m
11. off	40-60 min run	off	40-60 min run	25 min	off	16 miles
12. off	40-60 min run	off	40-60 min run	25 min	off	13 x 800m
13. off	40-60 min run	off	40-60 min run	25 min	off	19 miles
14. off	40-60 min run	off	40-60 min run	25 min	off	14 x 800m
15. off	40-60 min run	off	40-60 min run	25 min	off	4 miles
16. off	30-45 min run	off	30-45 min run	20 min	off	HM*
17. off	30-45 min run	off	30-45 min run	20 min	off	5 miles

* HM = Half marathon

8. Warm up for each 800-meter repeat workout by walking for 5 minutes, then jogging very slowly for 5-10 minutes. Then do 4-8 acceleration gliders (see the segment on drills in this book). Cool down at the end by jogging slowly for 5 minutes and then walking for 5 minutes. Walk 3 min between each 800-meter repeat. You may choose to run the 800s continuously or take a short walk break. At the end of the first lap, walk for 20-30 seconds but don't stop your stopwatch. The time for each 800 should be from the start until the end of the second lap.

9. If you have recovered from the weekend workout on Tuesday, run 3-4 "race rehearsal" miles (noted as "rr" on the Tue line). After an easy warm-up, run 4 of the cadence drills (CD) and 4 acceleration gliders (AG). These are described in the drill section of this book. Then run 3-4 x one mile (1600 meter) segments, taking the walk breaks as you plan to do them in the race. Jog for 1-2 minutes between these rr miles. Jog for the rest of your run. As the weeks pass, try various ratios of running/walking to see which feels best when running your goal pace.

10. It is fine to do cross-training on Monday, Wednesday, and Friday, if you wish. There will be little benefit to your running in doing this, but you'll increase your fat-burning potential. Don't do exercises like stair machines that use the calf muscle on these recovery days.

11. Be sure to take a vacation from strenuous exercise the day before your weekend runs.

12. On Thursday, run a few hill repeats (h) as described by the hill section in this book – except for the days set aside for the MMs.

TIME GOAL PROGRAM: 1:30-1:44

To find per kilometer pace, convert mile pace to a decimal and multiply by .62. For example, 10:24 per mile would be 10.4 x .62 = 6.448 which = 6:27/km.

Note: This is the minimum that I've found necessary to prepare for this goal. If you are already running more than this amount, and are able to recover between workouts, you may continue to do what you are doing – but be careful.

1. To begin this program, you should have run a long run within the past two weeks of at least 7 miles. If your long run is not this long, then gradually increase the weekend run to this distance before starting this program.

2. What is my current level of performance? Read the chapter in this book on "Choosing the Right Goal." After you run the first "Magic Mile" (MM), multiply by 1.2. This predicts what you what you are currently capable of running in a half marathon (per mile) right now, when the temperature is 60F or below, and if you have done the long runs and speed training listed in the schedule. If you want to improve, see the "Predicting Race Performance" section in this book.

3. What pace should I run on the long runs? Take your current performance level (MM x 1.2) and add 3 minutes – the result is your suggested long run pace per mile on long runs at 60F (14C)or cooler.

4. On long runs and the race itself, slow down when the temperature rises above 60F (14C) by 30 sec a mile for every 5 degrees above 60F or more (20 sec/km slower for every 2C above 14C).

5. Run-Walk-Run ratio should correspond to the pace used.

Mon	Tue	Wed	Thu	Fri	Sat	Sun
1. off	40-60 min run	off	40-60min (MM)	25 min	off	8 miles
2. off	40-60 min run	off	1 mi MM +3mi	25 min	off	5 x 800m
3. off	40-60 min run	off	40-60min (MM)	25 min	off	9.5 miles
4. off	40-60 min run	off	40-60min (MM)	25 min	off	7 x 800m
5. off	40-60 min run	off	40-60 min run	25 min	off	11 miles
6. off	40-60 min run	off	1 mi MM +4mi	25 min	off	9 x 800m
7. off	40-60 min run	off	40-60 min run	25 min	off	13 miles
8. off	40-60 min run	off	40-60 min run	25 min	off	11 x 800m
9. off	40-60 min run	off	40-60 min run	25 min	off	15 miles
10. off	40-60 min run	off	1 mi MM +4mi	25 min	off	12 x 800m
11. off	40-60 min run	off	40-60 min run	25 min	off	17 miles
12. off	40-60 min run	off	40-60 min run	25 min	off	13 x 800m
13. off	40-60 min run	off	40-60 min run	25 min	off	19 miles
14. off	40-60 min run	off	40-60 min run	25 min	off	14 x 800m
15. off	40-60 min run	off	40-60 min run	25 min	off	4 miles
16. off	30-45 min run	off	30-45 min run	20 min	off	HM*
17. off	30-45 min run	off	30-45 min run	20 min	off	5 miles

* HM = Half marathon

6. At the beginning of the program, after you have run the first MM, you can choose a goal that is as fast as 20 seconds per mile (15 sec/km) faster than predicted by the process indicated in number 2 in this section or any goal slower than this. To use this schedule, the goal pace should be between 7:00 and 8:00 per mile.

7. To compute your pace for the 800-meter (2 laps around a track) repeats done on speedwork weekends, take half the time of your goal pace per mile, as you decided according to number 6, and subtract 15 seconds. Example: for a 8 min/mi pace, run each 800 in 3:45.

8. Warm up for each 800-meter repeat workout by walking for 5 minutes, then jogging very slowly for 5-10 minutes. Then do 4-8 acceleration gliders (see the segment on drills in this book). Cool down at the end by jogging slowly for 5 minutes and then walking for 5 minutes. Walk 3 min between each 800-meter repeat. The time for each 800 should be from the start until the end of the second lap.

9.   If you have recovered from the weekend workout on Tuesday, run 4 "race rehearsal" miles (noted as "rr" on the Tue line). After an easy warm-up, run 4 of the cadence drills (CD) and 4 acceleration gliders (AG). These are described in the drill section of this book. Then run 3-4 x 1 mile (1600 meter) segments, taking the walk breaks as you plan to do them in the race. Jog for 1-2 minutes between these rr miles. Jog for the rest of your run. As the weeks pass, try various ratios of running/walking to see which feels best, running your goal pace.

10. It is fine to do cross-training on Monday, Wednesday, and Friday, if you wish. There will be little benefit to your running in doing this, but you'll increase your fat-burning potential. Don't do exercises like stair machines that use the calf muscle on these recovery days.

11. Be sure to take a vacation from strenuous exercise, the day before your weekend runs.

12. On Thursday, run a few hill repeats (h) as described by the hill section in this book – except for the days set aside for the MMs.

TIME GOAL PROGRAM: 1:15-1:29

To find per kilometer pace, convert mile pace to a decimal and multiply by .62. For example, 10:24 per mile would be 10.4 x .62 = 6.448 which = 6:27/km.

Note: This is the minimum that I've found necessary to prepare for the goal. If you are already running more than this amount, and are able to recover between workouts, you may continue to do what you are doing – but be careful.

1.   To begin this program, you should have run a long run within the past two weeks of at least 7 miles. If your long run is not this long, then gradually increase the weekend run to this distance before starting this program.

2.   What is my current level of performance? Read the chapter in this book on "Choosing the Right Goal." After you run the first "Magic Mile" (MM), multiply by 1.2. This predicts what you what you are currently capable of running in a half marathon (per mile) right now, when the temperature is 60F or below, and if you have done the long runs and speed training listed in the schedule. If you want to improve, see the "Predicting Race Performance" section in this book.

Mon	Tue	Wed	Thu	Fri	Sat	Sun
1. off	40-60 min run	off	40-60min (MM)	25 min	off	8 miles
2. off	40-60 min run	off	1 mi TT +3mi	25 min	off	5 x 800m
3. off	40-60 min run	off	40-60min (MM)	25 min	off	10 miles
4. off	40-60 min run	off	40-60 min run	25 min	off	7 x 800m
5. off	40-60 min run	off	40-60 min run	25 min	off	12 miles
6. off	40-60 min run	off	1 mi TT +4mi	25 min	off	9 x 800m
7. off	40-60 min run	off	40-60 min run	25 min	off	14 miles
8. off	40-60 min run	off	40-60 min run	25 min	off	11 x 800m
9. off	40-60 min run	off	40-60 min run	25 min	off	16 miles
10. off	40-60 min run	off	1 mi TT +4mi	25 min	off	12 x 800m
11. off	40-60 min run	off	40-60 min run	25 min	off	18 miles
12. off	40-60 min run	off	40-60 min run	25 min	off	13 x 800m
13. off	40-60 min run	off	40-60 min run	25 min	off	20 miles
14. off	40-60 min run	off	40-60 min run	25 min	off	14 x 800m
15. off	40-60 min run	off	40-60 min run	25 min	off	4 miles
16. off	30-45 min run	off	30-45 min run	20 min	off	HM*
17. off	30-45 min run	off	30-45 min run	20 min	off	5 miles

* HM = Half marathon

3. What pace should I run on the long runs? Take your current performance level (MM x 1.2) and add 3 minutes – the result is your suggested long run pace per mile on long runs at 60F (14C) or cooler.

4. On long runs and the race itself, slow down when the temperature rises above 60F (14C) by 30 sec a mile for every 5 degrees above 60F or more (20 sec/km slower for every 2C above 14C).

5. Run-Walk-Run ratio should correspond to the pace used.

6. At the beginning of the program, after you have run the first MM, you can choose a goal that is as fast as 20 seconds per mile (15 sec/km) faster than predicted by the process indicated in number 2 in this section or any goal slower than this. To use this schedule, the goal pace should be between 5:45 and 7:00 per mile.

7. To compute your pace for the 800-meter (2 laps around a track) repeats done on speedwork weekends, take half the time of your goal pace per mile, as you decided according to number 6, and subtract 15 seconds. Example: for a 7 min/mi pace, run each 800 in 3:15.

8. Warm up for each 800-meter repeat workout by walking for 5 minutes, then jogging very slowly for 5-10 minutes. Then do 4-8 acceleration gliders (see the segment on drills in this book). Cool down at the end by jogging slowly for 5 minutes and then walking for 5 minutes. Walk 3 min between each 800-meter repeat. The time for each 800 should be from the start until the end of the second lap.

9. If you have recovered from the weekend workout on Tuesday, run 4 "race rehearsal" miles (noted as "rr" on the Tue line). After an easy warm-up, run 4 of the cadence drills (CD) and 4 acceleration gliders (AG). These are described in the drill section of this book. Then run 3-4 x one mile (1600 meter) segments, taking the walk breaks as you plan to do them in the race. Jog for 1-2 minutes between these rr miles. Jog for the rest of your run. As the weeks pass, try various ratios of running/walking to see which feels best, running your goal pace.

10. It is fine to do cross-training on Monday, Wednesday, and Friday, if you wish. There will be little benefit to your running in doing this, but you'll increase your fat-burning potential. Don't do exercises like stair machines that use the calf muscle on these recovery days.

11. Be sure to take a vacation from strenuous exercise, the day before your weekend runs.

12. 12. On Thursday, run a few hill repeats (h) as described by the hill section in this book – except for the days set aside for the MMs.

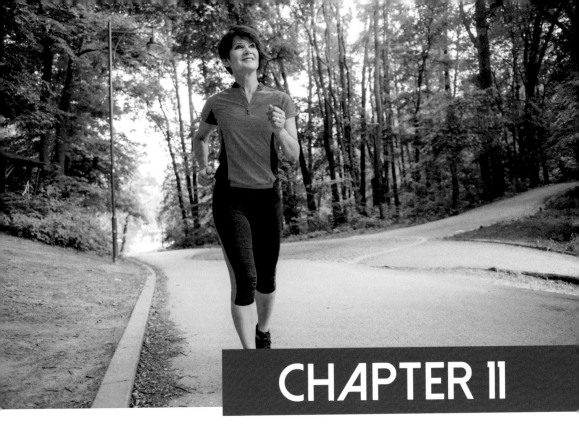

CHAPTER 11

THE DRILLS TO MAKE RUNNING FASTER AND EASIER

The following gentle drills, which were developed at my beach retreats and other individualized sessions, have helped thousands run more efficiently and faster. Each targets a few key capabilities. When you put all of them together, they can help you run lighter on your feet with better form while strengthening key muscle groups. When runners do these drills regularly, I've seen significant reduction of excess motion in feet and legs. Reduced impact running is easier when you run smoother and the improved cadence of your feet and legs can allow for faster running.

WHEN?

These should be done on a non-long-run day. It is fine, however, to do them as part of your warm-up before a race or a speed workout. Many runners have also told me that the drills are a nice way to break up an average run they sometimes call "boring." To receive a continuous benefit, they must be done once or twice every week.

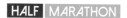
CADENCE DRILL (CD)

Everyone can benefit from doing the CD because it helps to pull all the elements of good running form together at the same time. Over the weeks and months, if you do this drill once every week, you will find that your normal cadence slowly increases naturally.

- Warm up by walking for 5 minutes, and running and walking very gently for 10 minutes.

- Start jogging slowly for 1-2 minutes and then time yourself for 30 seconds. During this half-minute, count the number of times your left or right foot touches (not both).

- Walk around for a minute or so.

- On the second 30-second drill, increase the count by 1 or 2.

- Repeat this 3-7 times. On each successive CD, try to increase by 1-2 additional steps.

- If you reach a count that you can't exceed, just try to maintain.

- Start each new CD with a blank slate. Whatever your count on the first one, just try to do more on the second.

In the process of improving cadence, the body's internal monitoring system coordinates a series of adaptations that makes the feet, legs, nervous system, and timing mechanism work together as an efficient team:

- Your foot touches more gently.

- Extra, inefficient motions of the foot and leg are reduced or eliminated.

- Less effort is spent on pushing up or moving forward.

- You stay lower to the ground.

- The ankle does most of the work, reducing leg muscle fatigue.

ACCELERATION GLIDER DRILLS (AG)

This drill will help you seamlessly transition from a walk into a run and then glide seamlessly back into a walk.

Note: Gliding is coasting off momentum as you gradually slow down into a "shuffle" and then a walk.

- Done on a non-long-run day, in the middle of a shorter run, or as a warm-up for a speed session or a race – or MM.
- Warm up with at least half a mile of easy running.
- Many runners do the CD just after the easy warm-up and then the AG. But the drills can be done separately also.
- Run 4-8 of them.
- Do this at least once a week.
- No sprinting – never run all-out.
- Don't do these if you have an injury.
- Stop immediately if you suspect that you are irritating a weak link.

After teaching this drill at my one-day running schools and weekend retreats for years, I can say that most people learn better through practice when they work on the following concepts (rather than the details of the drill). So just get out there and try them!

Gliding – The most important concept. This is like coasting off the momentum of a downhill run. You can do some of your gliders running down a hill if you want, but it is important to do at least two of them on flat land. Your goal is to use your momentum, if only for 5-10 strides, gliding for as many steps as you can.

Do this every week – As in the CDs, it's important to do them 1-2 times a week. If you're like most runners, you won't glide very far at first. Regular practice will help you glide farther and farther.

Don't sweat the small stuff – I've included a general guideline of how many steps to do with each part of the drill, but don't worry about getting an exact number of steps. It's best to get into a flow with this drill and not worry about how many steps you are taking.

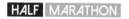

Smooth transition – Between each of the components. Each time you "shift gears," you are using the momentum of the current mode to start into the next mode. Don't make a sudden and abrupt change, but strive for a smooth transition between modes.

HERE'S HOW IT'S DONE:

- Each segment is about 8-10 steps except as noted in the following.
- Start with a walk.
- Ease into a shuffle (feet near the surface, baby steps, light touch).
- Ease into a slow jog.
- Ease into a normal pace on an easy day.
- If you will be running a MM race or a speed workout, then speed up gradually over about 30 steps to about the pace you'll be running. Note: No sprinting.
- Then glide or coast off momentum (you can extend the step count as needed to get a good glide).
- Ease into a shuffle.
- Ease into a walk.

Overall purpose: As you do this drill every week, you will feel smoother at each mode of running. Congratulations! You are learning how to keep moving at a fairly fast pace without using much energy. This is the main object of the drill. There will be some weeks when you will glide longer than others – don't worry about this. By doing this drill regularly, you will find yourself coasting or gliding down the smallest of inclines, and even for 10-20 yards on the flat, on a regular basis. Gliding conserves energy, reduces soreness and fatigue, and maintains a faster pace in races.

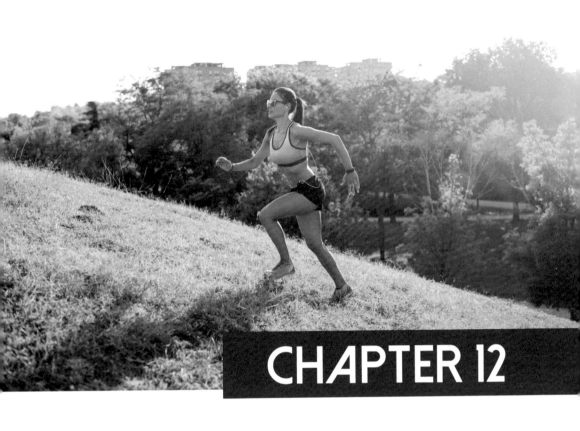

CHAPTER 12

HILL TRAINING BUILDS STRENGTH – AND MORE

Hill training strengthens the legs for running better than any other activity I know. At the same time, it can help you improve leg speed and enhance your ability to run hills in races. The hill training segments provide a gentle introduction to faster running, while improving your capacity to perform speedwork later in the program.

Beginners shouldn't do hill training. If you've run several road races, you could run 1-4 hills (as mentioned next) on one of the short runs during the week. More experienced runners can follow the scheduled hill sessions using the schedules in this book.

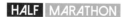

THE HILL WORKOUT

- Walk for 5 minutes.

- Warm-up: Jog and walk to a hill – about 10 minutes. Jog a minute and walk a minute (a longer warm up is fine).

- Do 4 acceleration gliders. These are listed in the "Drills" chapter (don't sprint).

- Walk 5-10 minutes as your cool-down.

- Choose a hill with a gentle grade – steep hills often cause problems and bestow no additional benefit.

- Walk to the top of the hill. Then step off the length of your hill segment by walking down from the top:

  - 50 walking steps for those new to hill training

  - 100-150 steps for those who have done very little speed work before

  - 150-200 steps for those who have done speedwork, but not within the past 6 months

  - 200-300 steps for those who have been doing regular speedwork

- Mark the place after you count the steps. This is where each hill starts.

- Run up the hill for 5 seconds, and then down for 5 seconds. Walk for 30-60 seconds. Repeat this 5-10 times. This finalizes the warm-up.

- Walk for 3-4 minutes.

- Run the first few steps of each hill acceleration at a jog, then gradually pick up the turnover of the feet as you go up the hill.

- Get into a comfortable rhythm so that you can gradually increase this rhythm or turnover (# of RPMs of feet and legs) as you go up the hill.

- Run with a relaxed stride and keep shortening stride as you go up the hill.

- It's OK to huff and puff at the top of the hill, but don't let the legs get overextended, or feel exhausted.

- Run over the top of the hill by at least 10 steps.

- Walk back to the top and keep walking for 1-2 minutes if you need to. Then run downhill, practicing good downhill form. Walk to recover before starting the next hill repeat.

HILL RUNNING FORM

- Start with a comfortable stride – fairly short.

- As you go up the hill, shorten the stride.

- Touch lightly with your feet.

- Maintain a body posture that is perpendicular to the horizon (upright, not leaning forward or back).

- Pick up the turnover of your feet as you go up and over the top.

- Keep shortening your stride so that the leg muscles don't tighten up; you want them as resilient as possible.

- Relax as you go over the top of the hill, and glide (or coast) a bit on the downside.

- It is OK to huff and puff as you go up the hill – no sprinting and no panting.

HILL TRAINING STRENGTHENS LOWER LEGS AND IMPROVES RUNNING FORM

The incline of the hill forces your legs to work harder as you go up. The extra work up the incline and the faster turnover builds strength. By taking an easy walk between the hills and an easy day afterward, the lower leg muscles become stronger.

Over several months, the improved strength allows you to support your body weight farther forward on your feet. An extended range of motion of the ankle and Achilles tendon results in a "bonus" extension of the foot forward with no increase in effort. You will run faster without working harder. What a deal!

RUNNING FASTER ON HILLS IN RACES

Once you train yourself to run with efficient hill form, you'll run faster with increased turnover on the hill workouts. This prepares you to do the same in races. You won't run quite as fast in a race as in your workouts. But through hill training, you can run faster than you used to run up the same hill on a race course.

Race hill technique is the same as in workouts: keep shortening stride as you move up the hill. Different from hill workouts is the strict monitoring of your respiration rate: don't huff and puff more than you were on the flat. As runners improve their hill technique in races, the general finding is that a shorter and quicker stride reduces effort while increasing speed with no increase in breathing.

> **Note:** On your long runs and easy running days, just jog up hills, don't run faster up the hill. If your breathing rate increases going up a hill, reduce effort and stride length, and take more frequent walk breaks until your respiration is as it was on the flat ground.

DOWNHILL FORM

- Run light on your feet.
- Maintain an average stride – avoid the temptation to extend stride.
- Keep feet low to the ground.
- Let gravity pull you down the hill.
- Cadence of the feet will pick up.
- Try to glide (or coast) quickly down the hill.
- You shouldn't have to use your quad muscles (front of thigh) by using this technique.

BIGGEST MISTAKES: TOO LONG A STRIDE, BOUNCING TOO MUCH

Even if the stride is one or two inches too long, your downhill speed can get out of control. If you are bouncing more than an inch or two off the ground, you run the risk of pounding your feet, having to use your quads to slow down (producing soreness), and creating shin and hamstring soreness due to overstriding. Tight hamstrings (big muscle behind your upper leg) are also a sign that you are overstriding.

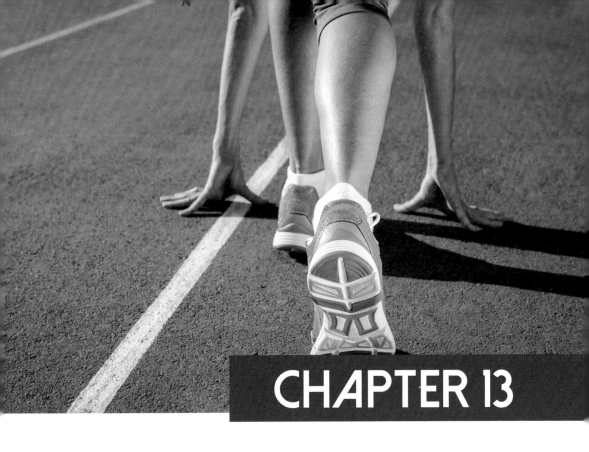

CHAPTER 13

SPEED TRAINING PREPARES YOU FOR TOP PERFORMANCE

At some point, virtually every runner wants to run a little faster. Often this desire is due to the envy of others who started when you did but have recorded faster finish times a year later. Beware! Some very sedentary people inherited a better set of fitness genes. Women are more at risk of injury from speed training and therefore need to be cautious. The leading cause of my time goal runners' injuries is speed training. This chapter will explain how speed training helps, and the internal changes that allow you to run faster while reducing injury risk.

I DON'T RECOMMEND TRAINING FOR A TIME GOAL IN YOUR FIRST HALF MARATHON

After you've finished your first campaign, come back to this chapter. During your first 21K training program, focus on the sense of satisfaction and achievement from continuing to push back your endurance through the long runs. Success is finishing.

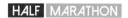

LEARN YOUR LIMITS

Most people go through their lives without ever testing their physical limits or experiencing the empowerment of extending them. Once into this process, some get swept away in the quest for improvement. When runners make speed-training mistakes, it is usually because they have done too much, too soon. The series of gentle increases through the training schedules in this book will gradually extend your capacity to go further at a slightly faster pace than you are running now.

Since each person can control the effort level, you will have a chance to limit or eliminate the damage. The adaptive process involves guessing and adjusting, going just a bit farther and then backing off. When done regularly, with sufficient rest between workouts, speed training prepares the mind, body, and spirit for greater challenges.

Each workout will provide a slight increase in the number of speed repetitions. At the same time you're improving muscle conditioning and cardiovascular performance, you'll gain pace judgement and mental toughness.

The overall experience of doing this, even for one season, progressively reduces race day anxiety as it develops confidence in confronting challenges in other areas of life. The best way I've found to prepare for pushing beyond your current "wall" in a fast race is to simulate the conditions during speed workouts.

BEWARE OF THE EGO

Some of the most timid beginning runners become overly aggressive competitors. As you find your times improving through regular training, the ego tells you what you want to hear. "If you improved 10 seconds with one weekly speed workout, then two hard workouts will double the improvement." Many runners have allowed their egos to mistakenly focus the satisfaction from finishing a run to the time on the finish line clock. This can reduce the wonderful enjoyment and satisfaction of a gentle run. An ego-driven runner loses the glow of endorphins when the watch tells them that they didn't run as fast as he/she "should." This line of thinking often leads to slower races (due to overtraining) and disappointment.

Even when times are improving, if time improvement is your primary reward from running, you'll often miss the enjoyment of an achievement on the way to the next time goal. My suggestion: take time to enjoy the best part of the run – the vitality and mental attitude boost.

It is healthy to let your ego have its moments of glory as you perform well. Just realize that improvement does not continue indefinitely. The ego has a problem with any downturn. A natural selection process occurs during a speed-training season, as the ego is forced to deal with reality and make adjustments. But by maintaining the enjoyment of a fun run every week and appreciating the afterglow from any run, you can maintain a balanced set of rewards, while keeping the ego in check.

While testing yourself for faster times can keep you focused and may increase motivation, the blending of mind, body, and spirit is maintained primarily through the enjoyment of the act of running. I've found that this is best done on slow runs, and in the slow warm-up and cool-down jogs that bracket your workouts. I've experienced an almost continuous stream of enjoyment from running for over half a century. It keeps getting better because I have regular doses of relaxing runs. Even when I was training for the Olympics, at least 80% of my weekly miles were spent running at a slow and enjoyable pace.

GETTING FASTER REQUIRES EXTRA WORK

To get faster, you must push beyond your current performance capacity. But you must be careful. Even a small amount over your speed limit can result in longer recovery or injury. The secret is to push only a little harder on each workout, then back off so the systems can rebound and improve. Gradual and gentle increases are always better because your body can adapt and you are more likely to sustain continuous and long-term improvement.

Our bodies are programmed to conserve resources by doing the smallest amount of work they can get away with. So even after we have increased the length of our runs steadily over several months, our leg muscles, tendons, ligaments, etc., are not prepared for the jolt that speed-training delivers. The best way to stay injury-free is to gradually increase the duration and intensity. But only when we put the legs, heart, lungs, etc., to a gentle test, week by week, does the body respond by improving:

- Mitochondria (energy powerhouses inside muscle cell) increase capacity and output

- Mechanical efficiency of the foot is improved – more work done with less effort

- Legs go further when tired – adaptations allow you to keep going

- Muscle cells work as a team – getting stronger, increasing performance, pumping blood back to the heart

- Mental concentration increases

- Your spirit is unleashed as you find yourself improving

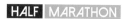

ENDORPHINS KILL PAIN, MAKE YOU FEEL GOOD

Running at any pace, but especially speed training, signals to your body that there will be some pain to kill. The natural response is to produce internal painkillers called endorphins. These hormones act as drugs tend to numb the exercising muscles while bestowing a good attitude – especially when you are tired after the run. Walk breaks reduce the stress on the system, reducing the need for killing pain, allowing these powerful positive attitude hormones to lock into receptor sites throughout the body/mind. You feel good!

GRADUALLY PUSHING UP THE WORKLOAD

Your body is programmed to improve when it is gradually introduced to a little more work with enough rest afterward. Push too hard or neglect the rest, and you'll see an increase in aches, pains, and injury. When speed workouts are balanced with rest afterward, adjustments are made to problems and goals are realistic, most runners can continue to improve for years.

REST ALLOWS YOUR BODY TO IMPROVE AFTER SPEEDWORK

When we run a little faster than our realistic goal pace and increase the number of repetitions a little more than we did on the last speed workout, this greater workload breaks down the muscle cells, tendons, etc., and stimulates change. Our bodies are programmed to rebuild stronger than before when slightly overwhelmed, if there is adequate rest after the harder workout.

INTRODUCING THE BODY TO SPEED THROUGH "DRILLS"

As a gentle introduction to faster running, I've found nothing better than the two drills that are detailed in the "Drills" chapter:

Cadence drills and acceleration gliders. The former helps to increase the number of steps per minute. The latter provides a very gentle introduction to speedwork, in very short segments. Most of the running during the conditioning period is at an easy pace. These drills, done in the middle of a short run once or twice a week, will improve mechanics, get the muscles ready for the heavier demands of speed training and initiate internal physiological changes in the muscles.

A GENTLE INCREASE IN SPEEDWORK CAUSES A SLIGHT BREAKDOWN

The speed workout starts with a few speed repetitions and rest between each. As the number of repetitions increases, your muscles are pushed slightly beyond the previous workout. With each extension, your conscious brain triggers circuits that drive muscle fibers to push past the previous maximum workload. They continue to perform like motivated workers to keep you running the pace assigned. In every session some are pushed beyond their capacity with each additional speed repetition. Often, pain and fatigue are not felt during the workout. But within one or two days, muscles, tendons, and joints can be sore with an overall feeling of fatigue. Even walking may not feel smooth for a day or two after a speed session that is run too hard. A little bit of these symptoms is fine. When you have a lot of it, you did too much. More than the average amount of tissue breakdown stimulates the release of cortisol, a repair hormone that has a depressive psychological effect.

THE DAMAGE

Looking inside the cell at the end of a hard workout, you'll see damage:

- Tears in the muscle cell membrane.

- The mitochondria (that process the energy inside the cell) are swollen.

- There's a significant lowering of the muscle stores of glycogen (the energy supply needed in speedwork).

- Waste products from exertion, bits of bone and muscle tissue and other bio junk can be found.

- Sometimes, there are small tears in the blood vessels and arteries, and blood leaks into the muscles.

THE DAMAGE STIMULATES THE MUSCLES, TENDONS, ETC., TO REBUILD STRONGER AND BETTER THAN BEFORE

Your body is programmed to get better when it is pushed beyond its current limits. A slight increase is better than a greater increase because the repair can be done relatively quickly.

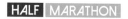

YOU MUST *HAVE* ENOUGH REST – IF YOU *WANT* TO REBUILD STRONGER *AND* BETTER

Two days after a speed session, if the muscles have had enough rest, you'll see some improvements:

• Waste has been removed.

• Thicker cell membranes can handle more work without breaking down.

• The mitochondria have increased in size and number, so that they can process more energy next time.

• The damage to the blood system has been repaired.

• Over several months, after adapting to a continued series of small increases, more capillaries (tiny fingers of the blood system) are produced. This improves and expands the delivery of oxygen and nutrients and provides a better withdrawal of waste products.

These are only some of the many adaptations made by the incredible human body when we do speedwork within current limits: biomechanics, nervous system, strength, muscle efficiency, and more. Internal psychological improvements follow the physical ones. Mind, body, and spirit are becoming a team, improving health and performance. An added benefit is a positive attitude.

QUALITY REST IS CRUCIAL: 48 HOURS BETWEEN WORKOUTS

On rest days, it's important to avoid exercises that strenuously use the calf muscle, ankle, and Achilles tendon (stair machines, step aerobics, spinning out of the saddle) for the 48-hour period between running workouts. If you have other aches and pains from your individual "weak links" then don't do exercises that could cause more aggravation.

Gentle walking is usually a great exercise for a rest day. There are several other good exercises in the "Cross-training" section of my books. Stay away from exercises that stress the calf muscle, feet, and ankle.

BEWARE OF JUNK MILES

Those training for a time goal often develop injuries because they try to "sneak in" a few miles on the days they should be resting. Even more than running long distance, speed training stresses the feet and legs and mandates the need for a 48-hour recovery period. The short, junk-mile days don't improve your conditioning, yet they prevent your muscles from recovering.

REGULARITY

To maintain the adaptations, you must regularly run about every 2 days. To maintain the speed improvements mentioned in this book, you should do the speed drills listed in the training schedules (acceleration gliders and cadence drills) and the speed repetitions every 2-3 weeks (the 800-meter speed sessions). It is OK to delay a workout every once in a while, but you need to stay on schedule as much as possible. Missing two workouts in a row will result in a slight loss in performance capacity. The longer you wait, the harder it will be to start up again.

"MUSCLE MEMORY"

Your neuromuscular system remembers the patterns of muscle activity that you have done regularly over an extended period of time. The longer you have been running regularly, the easier it will be to start up when you've had a layoff. During your first few months of speedwork, for example, if you miss a weekly workout, you will need to drop back a week and rebuild. But if you have run regularly for several years, and you miss a speed workout, little will be lost if you start the next one very slowly and ease into it. Be careful as you return to speed training if this happens.

AEROBIC RUNNING IS DONE DURING LONG RUNS

Aerobic means "in the presence of oxygen." This is the type of running you do when you feel "slow" and comfortable. When running aerobically, your muscles can get enough oxygen from the blood to process the energy in the cells (burning fat in most cases). The minimal waste products produced during aerobic running can be easily removed with no lingering build-up in the muscles.

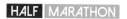

SPEED TRAINING GETS YOU INTO THE *ANAEROBIC* ZONE: *AN* OXYGEN DEBT

Anaerobic running means running so fast that your muscles can't get enough oxygen to burn the most efficient fuel, fat. So they shift to the limited supply of stored carbohydrate: glycogen. The waste products from this fuel pile up quickly in the cells, tightening the muscles and causing you to breathe heavily.

This is a clear sign of "oxygen debt." If you keep running for too long in this anaerobic state, you will have to slow down significantly or stop. But if you are running for a realistic time goal and are pacing yourself correctly, you should only be running anaerobically for a short period of time at the end of each workout and race.

THE *ANAEROBIC* THRESHOLD

As you increase the quantity of your speed sessions, you push back your anaerobic threshold. This means that you can run a bit farther than before (during each speed workout) without extreme huffing and puffing. Your muscles can move your body farther and faster without going to exhaustion. Each speed workout pushes you a little bit further into the anaerobic zone. Mind and body make adaptations to run farther before hitting a significant oxygen debt. You expand your capacity to simply keep going as the performance systems find a way to propel you even with waste products building up. The process of coping with the stress of speedwork is the essence of running faster.

THE TALK TEST - HOW *AEROBIC* ARE YOU?

- You're aerobic – if you can talk for as long as you want with minimal huffing and puffing (h & p).

- You are mostly aerobic – if you can talk for 30 sec + you cannot h & p for more than 10 sec.

- You are approaching anaerobic threshold – if you can only talk for 10 seconds or less, and then h & p for 10+ sec.

- You're anaerobic – if you can't talk more than a few words and are mostly huffing and puffing.

ARE YOU *WORKING* TOO HARD TOWARD A TIME GOAL?

When runners get too focused on specific time goals, the stress builds up and the subconscious reflex brain triggers negative hormones. At the first sign of these symptoms, back off a little and read the MENTAL TRAINING book for mantras and cognitive strategies that can shift control to the conscious brain. A strategy carried out by the conscious brain can keep you in charge and on a positive track.

OVERTRAINING STRESS SYMPTOMS

- Running is not as enjoyable.
- You don't look forward to your runs.
- When you say something to others about your running, the statements are often negative.
- The negativity can permeate other areas of your life.
- You look at running as work instead of play.

THE PERSONAL GROWTH OF SPEED TRAINING

Instead of looking at just the times in your races, embrace the life lessons that can come from the journey of an extended speed training program. Most of your runs must have some fun in them to help you through the challenges. Even after a hard workout, focus on how good you feel afterward and the satisfaction from overcoming the adversity.

Most runners find that speed training results in more setbacks than victories. But you'll learn more from the setbacks and they will make you a stronger runner and a stronger person. Confronting challenges is initially tough, but leads you to some of the great treasures of the improvement process. As runners dig deeper during speed sessions, they often find that they have more strength inside than was thought.

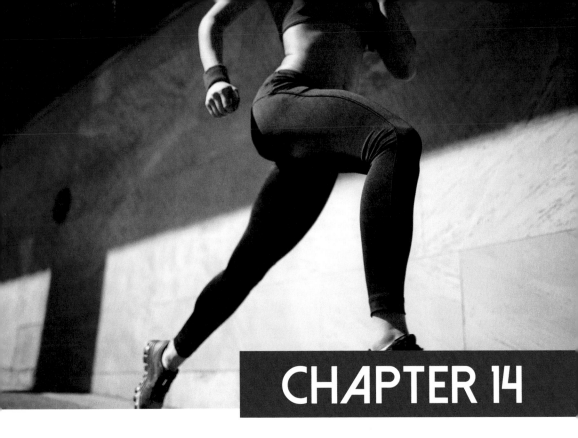

CHAPTER 14

HOW SPEED TRAINING WORKS

To run faster in the race, you need to run faster in some key workouts. The faster pace of both the workouts and the MMs challenge the mind/body to focus better and work at a higher level of performance: muscles, tendons, nerves, cardiovascular system, psyche, spirit. The regularity of the workouts sets up a process that consistently improves efficiency. You'll also search for and find new resources needed to deal with challenges not faced before.

800-METER REPEATS ARE RUN 15 SECONDS FASTER THAN HALF-MILE GOAL PACE

You'll see in the time goal schedules a series of 800-meter workouts on non-long-run weekends. These are best done on a track (two laps). Each should be run 15 seconds faster than you'd like to run half a mile in your goal race. Walk for the amount recommended in the training schedules.

KEEP GOING WHEN TIRED – THROUGH AN INCREASE IN THE NUMBER OF REPETITIONS

The maximum benefit from speed sessions is at the end of the program. As you increase the number of 800-meter speed repetitions from 4 to 6 to 8 and beyond, you teach yourself how to keep going at your assigned pace, even when tired. The only way I've found to prepare for this "race reality" situation is to keep pushing the envelope during speed training.

LONGER RUNS MAINTAIN ENDURANCE – AND IMPROVE YOUR TIME

Your long runs will maintain or extend endurance while you improve race finish time. Every week or two, you'll run a very slow longer run. Many surveys show that half marathoners improve their times as much or more by lengthening the long run as from speed training. To receive maximum improvement follow the schedules in this book and include both.

RUNNING FORM IMPROVES

Regular speed workouts stimulate your body to run more efficiently. On each workout, as you push into fatigue, your mind/body intuitively searches for ways of continuing to move at the same pace without extraneous motion: lighter touch of the feet, direct foot lift, lower to the ground, quicker turnover. See the running form chapter for more details.

WATCH OUT! SPEEDWORK INCREASES ACHES, PAINS, AND INJURIES

Speed training increases your chance of injury. Be sensitive to the areas on your foot, leg, muscles, etc., where you've had problems before – your weak links. Think back to the patterns of aches and pains that have caused you to reduce or stop exercise in the past. You can reduce injury risk significantly by taking a day or two off at the flare-up of one of these and by following the tips in the "troubleshooting injuries" section in this book.

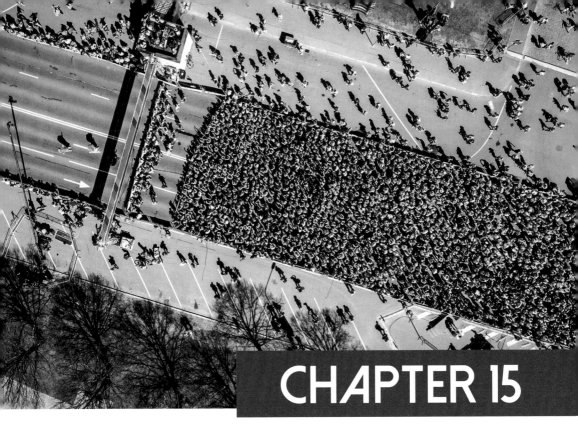

CHAPTER 15

RACE DAY TIMETABLE

Most runners who arrive at their first half marathon are surprised at the upbeat atmosphere. If the energy could be put in a container and used in your car, you wouldn't have to buy gasoline for weeks. Almost everyone at a race is in a good mood, and the shared excitement and optimism of the start continues joyously through the after-race party.

If it's your first race, look for one that:

- Is fun

- Has refreshments

- Has a T-Shirt and other goodies

- Entertainment

- The organizers focus on average or beginning runners

FASTER?

If you have run a half marathon and want to run faster, here are some other factors to consider:

- Difficulty of the course – ask your resources (next section) about this. Pick a course that tends to produce fast times.

- Weather conditions – look at the average temperatures for the day on which the race is scheduled to be below 60F. Remember that for every 5 degrees above 60F, you will tend to slow down by 30 sec a mile.

- Well organized – the organizers keep things organized: accurate measurement, accurate timing (usually using "the chip" technology), no long lines, easy to register, start goes off on time, water on the course, refreshments for all (even the slowest), no major problems.

- Competitive runners like the event and respect the organizers.

- How crowded? Half marathons that have more than about 15,000 runners often force runners to run half a mile farther than race distance. There are also bottlenecks that slow the pace.

RESOURCES: WHERE TO FIND OUT ABOUT RACES

RUNNING STORES

This resource is at the top of our list because you can usually get entry forms plus some editorial comment about the race. Explain to the store folks that this is your first race, or you're going for a fast time. Select a fun event that has a high rating in the "what to look for" section.

FRIENDS WHO RUN

Call a friend who has run for several years. Tell him or her that you are looking for a fun, upbeat race. Go over the same categories previously listed. Be sure to ask the friend for a contact number or website where you can find more information on the event, and possibly enter. As with running store folks, the editorial comments and evaluation of an event can steer you to a good experience.

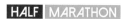

RUNNING CLUBS

If there is a running club or two in your area, get in touch. The officers or members can steer you in the direction of events. Running clubs may be found by doing a web search: type "running clubs (your town)." The RRCA (Road Runner's Club of America) is a national organization of neighborhood clubs. From their website, search for a club in your area.

NEWSPAPER LISTINGS

In many newspapers, there is a listing of community sports events, in the weekend section. This comes out on Friday or Saturday in most cities, usually in the lifestyle section. Some listings can be in the sports section under "running" or "road races." You can often find these listings on the website of the newspaper.

WEB SEARCHES

Just do a web search for "road races (your town)" or "5K (your town)." There are several event companies that serve as a registration center for many races: including *www.marathonguide.com* and *www.active.com*. From these sites, you can sometimes find an event in your area, research it, and then sign up. I recommend races I know about in my free newsletter. Sign up at *www.JeffGalloway.com*.

Note: Come to my Half Marathon (and Barb's 5K) in Atlanta for Galloway pace groups, fun, great medals, and more. I will be at the finish until the last person crosses.

RUNDISNEY EVENTS = GREAT FUN!

The Disney folks know how to facilitate events and make them fun. These events are spread throughout the year at Walt Disney World and Disneyland. The women-oriented events have been embraced by women who bring mothers, daughters, roommates, and families for a great weekend experience: Princess Half Marathon at WDW and Tinkerbell Half Marathon at Disneyland. I have also provided training programs for all of their events, including the Wine & Dine Half Marathon, Tower of Terror 10 mile, and Walt Disney World Marathon with video clips of my drills and other training components on the site: www.runDisney.com.

THE DONNA MARATHON: FINISH BREAST CANCER

This Jacksonville Beach, Florida, event is held in February. Almost every penny of the entry fee goes to breast cancer research at Mayo Clinic/care for women. The community supports this event, and the crowds are great. Scenic course, Galloway pace groups, and an upbeat weekend make this a great destination. There's a 7-hour limit on the half marathon, so walkers can win their medal here.

HOW TO REGISTER - ENTER EARLY!

More and more of the fun races are closing registration early because of increased demand. As soon as you have made the decision and coordinated with key family members or friends, sign up.

- **Online.** Most of the desirable events are conducting registration online. This allows you to bypass the process of finding an entry form and sending it in before the deadline.

- **Fill out an entry and send it in.** You will need to fill out your name, address, T-shirt size, etc., and then sign the waiver form. Be sure to include a check for the entry fee. Make sure that this is allowed and you are within the timeframe for registration.

- **Show up on race day.** Because some races don't do race day registration, be sure this is allowed. There is usually a penalty for waiting until the last minute, but you can see what the weather is like before you make the trek to the race.

REHEARSAL

If at all possible, run one or more of your long runs on the race course. You'll learn how to get there, where to park (or which rapid transit station to exit), and what the site is like. If you will be driving, drive into the parking area several times to make sure you understand exactly how to go where you need to park. This will help you to feel at home with the staging area on race day. Run over the last half-mile of the course at least twice. This is the most important part of the course for mental focus. It's also beneficial to do the first part of the course to see which side of the road is best for walk breaks (sidewalks, etc.).

Visualize your line up position. First-time half marathoners should line up at the back. If you line up too far forward you could slow down runners who are faster. You want to do this first race slowly and have a good experience. This is most likely at the back of the pack. Because you will be taking your walk breaks, as in training, you need to stay at the side of the road. If there is a sidewalk, you can use this for your walk breaks.

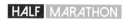

Tip: Line up at the back of your corral. In many of the races that are timed by computer chips, it helps to line up at the back of your corral. When the corral is released, wait for the other runners to get ahead by about a minute or so. When you start running and cross the start line, your timing clock starts and you have some space to run for a while.

THE AFTERNOON BEFORE

Don't run the day before the race. You won't lose any conditioning if you take two days off from running leading up to the race. If the race has an expo or other festivities, this is often interesting. Companies in the running business have displays, shoes, clothing, books, etc. – often at sale prices. Beware of sale shoes, however. It is best to go to a good running store and go through the procedure noted in my book to select a shoe that is designed for the type of foot you have.

Some races require you to pick up your race number and sometimes your computer chip (explained next) the day before. Look at the website or the entry form for instructions about this. Most races don't allow you to pick up your materials on race day, but be sure.

RACE NUMBER

This is sometimes called a "bib number." It should be pinned on the front of the garment you'll be wearing when you cross the finish line.

COMPUTER CHIP

More and more races are using technology that electronically records your race number and time as you cross the finish. You must wear this chip that is usually laced on the shoes, near the top. Some companies have a velcro band that is attached to the ankle or arm. Read the instructions to make sure you are attaching this correctly. Be sure to turn this in after the race. The officials have volunteers to collect them, so stop and take them off your shoe, etc. There is often a steep fine for those who don't turn in the chip.

THE CARBO-LOADING DINNER

Some races have a dinner the night before where you can chat with runners at your table and enjoy the evening. Don't over eat! Many runners assume, mistakenly, that they must "load up" the night before, which is actually counterproductive. It takes at least 24 hours for most of the food you eat to be processed and useable in a race – usually longer. If your blood sugar level is low, be sure to eat just enough to keep it adequately balanced. The downside is that too much "loading" the night before can lead to "unloading" during the long run the next day.

While you don't want to starve yourself the afternoon and evening before, the best strategy is to eat small meals, and taper down the amount as you get closer to bed time. As always, it's best to have done a "rehearsal" of eating so that you know what works, how much, when to stop eating, and what foods to avoid.

The evening before your long run is a good time to work on your eating plan and replicate the successful routine leading up to race day.

DRINKING

The day before, drink about 6 x 8oz of water and two glasses of a good electrolyte beverage like Accelerade. When you wake up on race morning, drink a 6 oz glass of water or a cup of coffee as soon as you can after rising. The more you drink after this, the more likely you will have to take toilet stops during the race itself. Many races have porto-johns around the course, but some do not. It is a very common practice for runners who have consumed too much fluid that morning to find a tree or alley along the course.

RULE OF THUMB FOR DRINKING DURING THE RACE:

2-4 oz of water every 2 miles.

Tip: If you practice drinking during your long runs, you can find the right amount of fluid that works best for you on race day. Don't drink more than 20 oz an hour.

THE NIGHT BEFORE

Eating is optional after 6pm. If you are hungry, have a light snack that you have tested before and has not caused problems. Less is better, but don't go to bed hungry.

Alcohol is not generally recommended because the effects of this central nervous system depressant carry over to the next morning. Some runners have no trouble having one glass of wine or beer, while others are better off with none. If you decide to have a drink, I suggest that you make it one portion.

Pack your bag and lay out your clothes so that you don't have to think very much on race morning.

- Your watch

- Your run/walk/run timer, set up for your strategy

- Shoes

- Socks

- Shorts

- Top – see clothing thermometer

- Pin race bib on the front of the garment in which you will be finishing

- A few extra safety pins

- Water, Accelerade, pre-race and post-race beverages (such as Endurox R4), and a cooler if you wish

- Food for the drive in and the drive home

- Bandages, Vaseline, any other first aid items you may need

- Cash for registration if you are doing race day registration (check for exact amount, including late fee)

- $25-40 for gas, food, parking, etc.

- Race chip attached according to the race instructions

- A few jokes or stories to provide laughs or entertainment before the start

- A copy of the "race day checklist"

SLEEP

You may sleep well, or you may not. Don't worry about it if you don't sleep at all. Many runners I work with every year don't sleep at all the night before and have the best race of their lives. Of course, don't try to go sleepless but if it happens, it's usually the worry and not the sleep deprivation that lowers performance.

RACE DAY CHECKLIST

Photocopy this list so that you will not only have a plan, but you can carry it out in a methodical way. This empowers the conscious brain to take control and reduce or eliminate anxious and negative hormones from the subconscious brain. Pack the list in your race bag. Don't try anything new the day of your race except for health or safety reasons. The only item I have heard about when used for the first time in a race that has helped is walk breaks. Even first- time users benefit significantly. Otherwise, stick with your plan.

Fluid and potty stops – After you wake up, drink 6 oz of water or coffee and then wait until you are running. If you have used Accelerade about 30 minutes before your runs, prepare it. Use a cooler if you wish. In order to avoid the bathroom stops, stop your fluid intake according to what has worked for you before.

Food – Eat what you have eaten before your harder runs. It is OK not to eat at all before a half marathon unless you are a diabetic, then go with the plan that you and your doctor (or nutritionist) have worked out.

Get your bearings – Walk around the site to find where you want to line up (at the back of the pack or in a pace group) and how you will get to the start. Choose a side of the road that has more shoulder or sidewalk for ease in taking walk breaks.

Register or pick up your race number – If you already have all of your materials, you can bypass this step. If not, look at the signage in the registration area and get in the right line. Usually there is one for "race day registration" (when offered) and one for those who registered online or in the mail and need to pick up their numbers.

Start your warm-up 40-50 min before the start. If possible, go backwards on the course for about .5-.6 mi and turn around. This will give you a preview of the most important part of your race – the finish.

Here is the warm-up routine:

- Walk for 5 minutes, slowly

- Walk at a normal walking pace for 3-5 minutes, with a relaxed and short stride

- Set your timer for the ratio of running and walking that you are using and do this for 10 minutes

- Walk around for 5-10 minutes

- If you are shooting for a time goal, do 4-8 acceleration gliders

- If you have time, walk around the staging area, read your jokes, laugh, relax

- Get in position and pick one side of the road or the other where you want to line up

- When the road is closed and runners are called to line up, go to the curb and stay at the side of the road, near or at the back of the crowd (for first-timers)

AFTER THE START

Remember that you can control how you feel during and afterward by conservative pacing and walk breaks.

Stick with the run/walk ratio that has worked for you – take every walk break, especially the first one.

- If it is warm, slow down and walk more (30 sec/mi slower for every 5F increase in temperature above 60/ 20 sec/km for every 2C increase above 14C)

- Don't let yourself be pulled out too fast on the running portions

- As people pass you who don't take walk breaks, tell yourself that you will catch them later – you will

- If anyone interprets your walking as weakness, say: "This is my proven strategy for a strong finish"

- Talk with folks along the way, enjoy the course, smile often

- On warm days, pour water over your head at the water stops (no need to drink on a 5K unless you want to)

AT THE FINISH

- In the upright position
- With a smile on your face
- Wanting to do it again

AFTER THE FINISH

- Keep walking for at least half a mile
- Drink about 4-8 oz of fluid
- Within 30 min of the finish, have a snack that is 80% carbohydrate/20% protein (Endurox R4 is best)
- If you can soak your legs in cool water during the first two hours after the race, do so for 10-20 min
- Walk for 20-30 minutes later in the day

THE NEXT DAY

- Walk for 30-60 minutes, very easy; this can be done at one time, or in installments
- Keep drinking about 4-6 oz an hour of water or sports drink like Accelerade
- Wait at least a week before you either schedule your next race or vow to never run another one again

CHAPTER 16

YOUR JOURNAL WILL INSPIRE YOU

"Journals give us control over our future while they allow us to learn from our past."

It would be wonderful if we never had to write anything down. In this magical world, you could rely upon your brain to track and retain everything you do, and constantly sort it to prepare you for the next few activities. Then, moments before you were scheduled to do something, a brain transmission would arrive, telling you exactly what to do, where to do it, the materials you need, and the deadline. And while we're dreaming, this would be done with complete consistency, hour after hour, day after day.

Since we don't operate in a perfect world, with a perfect brain, a journal allows us to activate the executive brain in the frontal lobe. This is the center for planning, strategy, scheduling, analyzing, articulating lessons learned, and charting our progress in a consistent direction. Your journal is actually a tool that will activate the conscious brain that can manage the emotional rollercoaster that may come from the subconscious brain under stress. With a simple logbook format that each of us chooses, we can see what to do, usually within a few minutes and make the adjustments necessary.

I'm not suggesting that everything be scheduled in advance. Some of the most inspiring moments and memorable actions sneak up on us unexpectedly. In your journal, you can trap these and relive the positive feelings. But by using your journal to plan ahead, you're programming the brain to continuously steer toward interesting opportunities that arise as you fine-tune the training and the goal. You don't even have to have a time goal to benefit from a journal. Journals are extremely helpful in ensuring that you schedule and record the rest you need for rebuilding and the enjoyable components that motivate us, while avoiding the stressful trends that produce injury.

Of all the activities that surround running, it is the writing and review of your journal that bestows the greatest control over the direction of your training. It only takes a few minutes every other day to record the key information. Looking back through your entries will provide laughs and enjoyment. You'll revisit the interesting things you saw during the last week, the crazy thoughts, the people you met and the fun. This process can inspire the frontal lobe's right brain to produce more entertainment as you schedule runs that deliver more fun.

JOURNAL KEEPERS ARE MORE LIKELY TO BE LIFELONG RUNNERS

Many beginning runners tell me that the writing of each day's mileage in the journal was the main reason they continued running during the first year – simple but satisfying. After a few weeks, many runners learn the empowerment of organizing runs in the journal. By the time 6 months have passed, you'll discover the satisfaction of looking back to chart progress while looking ahead several months to schedule races, training, and fun events along the way. I hear from several runners every month who use their journal as a diary of their life, noting other significant activities, their kids' soccer scores, and PTA notes.

It's a fact that those who journal their running, tend to run more days per year. The journal becomes the steering wheel that keeps you on the road of positive progress. As you hold tight and use the wheel, you feel an empowering sense of making progress – you and your conscious brain are in control.

RESTORING ORDER

One runner told me, "When my spouse died, and my life seemed to be in chaos, I felt a simple and powerful sense of security in documenting the distance that I covered each day. No one could take that away from me." Another runner commented, "As a young executive and a young mom, I felt that I had no control over my life until I started using

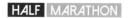

a training journal. It started with writing distance, then temperature, pace and route. My journal writing time was the only part of my day when I felt I had control. It was wonderful!"

A SIMPLE REWARD CAN PULL YOU OUT OF THE DUMPS

We all feel better and enjoy our activities when we feel rewarded. The simple act of recording the distance you cover each day will give you a genuine sense of accomplishment that is felt internally. When you string together a series of runs on days you didn't feel like running, you feel so good inside. Even the most upbeat people have periods of low motivation and have told me that their journals got them re-focused on the down days.

THIS IS YOUR BOOK

Yes, you are writing a book. At the most basic level, you will have an outline of your running life during the next few months. No one tells you what goes into this book. As runners record their entries in the log, they realize that they can use the same journal to organize other areas of life. Even runners who are not fired up about the process at first are usually impressed at how many benefits come from using this tool. Since you don't need to show anyone your journal, you can let your feelings flow as you write. Upon review, your emotional response to a given workout can be very interesting months or years later.

CAN YOU CAPTURE THE FLEETING THOUGHTS OF THE RIGHT BRAIN?

One of the interesting challenges, and great rewards of journaling, is noting the creative and sometime crazy images that emerge from the right side of our frontal lobe. On some days, you won't get any of these, and on others, the faucet opens up. Often the thoughts come out of nowhere. Other times, you will be suddenly hit with a solution to a problem you've been working on for months. If you have your journal available at the place where you return from your run – car, office desk, kitchen countertop – you can quickly jot some key words to describe the images or craziness.

Week of | Jan 1

Thursday

GOAL	35 min easy (SC)
TIME	45 min
DISTANCE	@ 6.5
AM PULSE	49
WEATHER	Cloudy
TEMP	40°
TIME	6 — AM/PM
TERRAIN	rolling
DATE	Jan 4
WALK BREAK	—

COMMENTS

1 2 3 4 5 6 ⑧ 9 10

Great run with Barb, Wes + Sambo — who took out the pace too fast + died at the end. The rest of us caught up on the gossip. Achilles ached so I iced it for 15 minutes.

Friday

GOAL	45 min (SP) 5 × 800 meter
TIME	1:15
DISTANCE	7.5 mi
AM PULSE	53
WEATHER	45°
TEMP	Sunny
TIME	5 — AM/PM
TERRAIN	track
DATE	Jan 5
WALK BREAK	400 m

COMMENTS

1 2:30
2 2:36
3 2:33
4 2:37
5 felt
6
7 Perform 2:32
8 2:36
9
10

My best workout in years!
- walked 400m between each
- struggled on last one

Achilles ached - iced 15 min

12 min warm up and warm down

Saturday

GOAL	Off
TIME	
DISTANCE	
AM PULSE	55
WEATHER	
TEMP	
TIME	AM/PM
TERRAIN	
DATE	Jan 6
WALK BREAK	

COMMENTS

1 2 3 4 5 6 7 8 9 10

Kids soccer (Morn)
* Westin scores goal bouncing off his back
  1st goal of season!
Brennan's cross country (aft)
     Invitational
* Brennan comes from 8th to 3rd in the last half mile. I'm so proud!

Sunday

GOAL	18 mi (1) easy!
TIME	2:53
DISTANCE	18 mi
AM PULSE	52
WEATHER	50°
TEMP	dry no wind
TIME	— AM/PM
TERRAIN	flat
DATE	Jan 7
WALK BREAK	1 min / mi

COMMENTS

1 2 3 4 5 ⑥ 7 8 9 10

It was great to cover 18 miles — wish I had a group
longest run in 18 months!
     but...
* went too fast in the first 5 miles
* Achilles hurt afterward - take 3 days off
* Power Bar + water from 10 mi kept spirits up

* Pulse is up — I'm not recovering — need more days off/week

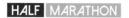

THE VARIOUS TYPES OF JOURNALS

Calendar – facing you on the wall

Many runners start recording their runs on a wall calendar – or one that is posted on the refrigerator. Looking at the miles recorded is empowering. But equally motivating for many is seeing too many "zeros" on days that should have been running days. If you're not sure whether you will really get into this journal process, you may find it easiest to start with a calendar.

AN ORGANIZED RUNNING JOURNAL

When you use a product that is designed for running, you don't have to think to record the facts. The spaces on the page ask you for certain info, and you will learn to fill it very quickly. This leaves you time to use some of the open space for the creative thoughts and ideas that pop up during a run. Look at the various journals available and pick one that looks easier to use and carry with you. I've included a sample page of my training journal as one example.

NOTEBOOK

You don't need to have a commercial product. You can create your own journal by using a basic school notebook of your choice. Find one in a size that works best with your lifestyle (briefcase, purse, etc.). Below you will find the items that I've found helpful to record. But the best journals are those that make it easier for you to collect the data you find interesting while allowing for creativity. The non-limiting nature of a notebook is a more comfortable format for runners who like to write a lot one day and not so much another day.

COMPUTER LOGS

There are a growing number of software products that allow you to sort through information more quickly. This format speeds up the search for information you need. As you set up your own codes and sections you can pick data that is important to you, sort it to see trends, and plan ahead. Some software allows for you to download data from a heart monitor or GPS watch.

THE *W*RITING PROCESS

- ## Capturing the flow from the right brain

  Try to have the log handy so that you can record info after a run. Immediately after a run, you will have fresh perceptions, and will be more likely to record the right brain images and thoughts that tend to fade quickly.

- ## Just the facts

  At first, spend a few seconds and quickly jot down the key info that you want recorded. If you have to think about an item, skip it and just fill in the items you can fill in quickly. Here is a list of items that many runners use:

Date:

Morning pulse:

Time of run:

Distance covered:

Time running:

Weather:

Temperature:Precipitation:Humidity:

Walk-Run frequency:

Any special segments of the run (speed, hills, race, etc.):

Running companion:

Terrain:

How did you feel (1-10):

Comments:

Go back over the list again and fill in more details – emotional responses, changes in energy or blood sugar level, and location of places where you had aches and pains, even if they went away during the run. You are looking for patterns of items that could indicate injury, blood sugar problems, lingering fatigue, etc.

- Helpful additions (usually in a blank section at the bottom of the page)
- Improvement thoughts
- Things I should have done differently
- Interesting happenings
- Funny things
- Strange things
- Stories, right brain crazy thoughts

ARE YOU TIRED ... OR JUST LAZY? YOUR MORNING PULSE MAY TELL

Many people say that they are too tired to run. But after interviewing many who make this claim, I've come to believe that the most common cause is laziness (most will admit this). A secondary cause is low blood sugar. If you have trained too hard, the best indicator I've found is resting pulse taken in the morning. Your journal can track this (although some runners use a piece of graph paper).

RECORDING MORNING PULSE

- As soon as you are conscious, but before you have thought much about anything, count your pulse rate for a minute. Record it before you forget it. If you don't have your journal by your bed, then keep a piece of paper handy with a pen.

- It is natural for there to be some fluctuation, based on the time you wake up, how long you have been awake, etc. But after several weeks and months, these will balance themselves out. The ideal would be to catch the pulse at the instant that you are awake, before you are hit with the shock of an alarm clock, thoughts of work stress, etc..

- After 2 weeks or so of readings, you can establish a baseline morning pulse. Take out the top 2 high readings and then compute an average.

- The average is your guide. If the rate is 5% higher than your average, take an easy day. When the rate is 10% higher, and there is no reason for this (you woke up from an exciting dream, medication, infection, etc.) then your muscles may be indeed tired. Take the day off if you have a run scheduled for that day.

If your pulse stays high for more than a week, call your doctor to see if there is a reason for this (medication, infection, hormones, metabolic changes, etc.).

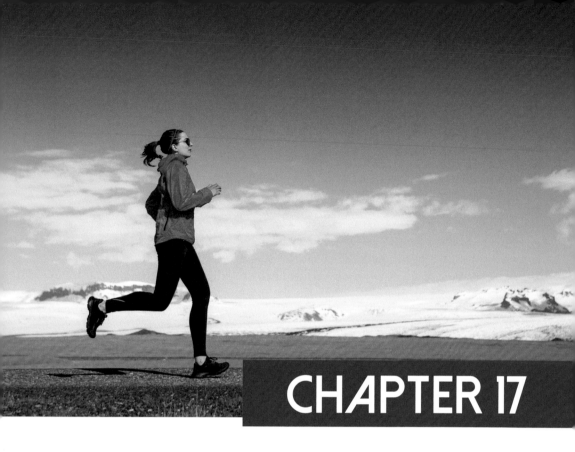

CHAPTER 17

RUNNING FORM

I believe that running is an inertia activity: your mission is simply to run smoothly and maintain momentum. Very little strength is needed to run. The first few strides get you into motion, and your focus thereafter is to stay in motion. To reduce fatigue, aches, and pains, your body intuitively fine tunes your motion so that you minimize effort as you continue to run month after month.

Humans have many biomechanical adaptations for running and walking, which have been made more efficient for more than a million years. The anatomical origin of efficiency in humans is the combination of the calf muscle, ankle, and the Achilles tendon. This is an extremely sophisticated system of levers, springs, balancing devices, and more, involving hundreds of components amazingly well coordinated. Biomechanics experts believe that this degree of development was not needed for walking. When our ancient ancestors had to run to survive, evolution reached a new level of performance.

When a runner develops efficient running form and uses the right balance of walking and running, very little effort from the calf muscle produces a smooth continuation of forward movement. As the calf muscle gets in better shape, and you apply the right run/walk/run strategy, you can keep going, mile after mile, with little perceived effort. Other muscle groups offer support and fine tune the process.

When you feel aches and pains that might be due to the way you run, going back to the minimal use of the ankle and Achilles tendon can often leave you feeling smooth and efficient very quickly.

Reducing stride length and staying low to the ground will reduce effort and injury risk. This motion relies on the ankle and reduces fatigue in the calf muscle – the main reason why runners slow down at the end of races. Read more about this next.

A BETTER WAY OF RUNNING?

There may be a better way for you to run, one that will leave your legs with more strength and result in fewer aches and pains. The fact is, however, that most runners are not far from great efficiency. Repeated research on runners has shown that most are running very close to their ideal. I believe this is due to the action of the right brain. After tens of thousands of steps, it keeps searching for (and then refines) the most efficient pattern of feet, legs, and body alignment.

In my full-day running schools and weekend retreats, I conduct an individual running form analysis with each runner. After having analyzed over ten thousand runners, I've also found that most are running in a very efficient way. The problems are seldom big ones, but a series of small mistakes. By making a few minor adjustments, most runners can feel better on every run.

THE BIG THREE: POSTURE, STRIDE, AND BOUNCE

In these consultations, I've also discovered that when runners have problems, they tend to occur in three areas: posture, stride, and bounce. And the problems tend to be individual in nature. They occur most often in specific areas because of specific motions. Fatigue increases the irritation of the "weak link" areas. A slight overstride, for example, creates fatigue and then a feeling of weakness at the end of a run. As a tired body "wobbles," other muscle groups try to keep the body on course but are not designed for this.

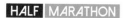
FOUR NEGATIVE RESULTS OF INEFFICIENT FORM

1. Fatigue becomes so severe that it takes much longer to recover.

2. Muscles are pushed so far beyond their limits that they break down and become injured.

3. The experience is so negative that the desire to run is reduced, producing burnout.

4. The "weak links" in your body become over-used and break down.

I've not seen anyone run with perfect form, which is specific to the individual anyway. I don't suggest that everyone should try to run perfectly because we have many adaptations based upon our unique range of motion. But when you become aware of your form problems and make changes to keep them from producing aches and pains, you'll experience fewer aches, smoother running, and faster times. This chapter can help you understand why aches and pains tend to come out of form problems and how you may be able to reduce or eliminate them. Be sure to read the section at the end of the book on troubleshooting aches and pains.

IF YOU FEEL RELAXED AND RUNNING IS EASY EVEN AT THE END OF A RUN, YOU'RE PROBABLY RUNNING CORRECTLY

Overall, the running motion should feel smooth, relaxed, and easy most of the time. There should be no tension in your neck, back, shoulders, or legs. If you are experiencing some issues of this type, posture or foot/leg placement are often the cause. Don't try to run through tightness or pain, try to adjust your running motion (with a few more walk breaks) so that the symptoms go away.

POSTURE

Good running posture is actually good body posture. The head is naturally balanced over the shoulders, which are aligned over the hips. As the foot comes underneath, all of these elements are in balance so that no energy is needed to prop up the body. You shouldn't have to work to pull a wayward body back from a wobble or inefficient motion.

FORWARD LEAN

The posture errors tend to be mostly due to a forward lean – especially when we are tired. The head wants to get to the finish as soon as possible, but the legs can't go any faster. In their first races, beginners are often the ones whose heads are literally ahead of the body, which produces more than a few falls around the finish line. A forward lean will often concentrate fatigue, pain, and tightness in the lower back or neck.

It all starts with the head. When the neck muscles are relaxed, the head is usually in a natural position. If there is tension in the neck, or soreness afterward, the head is usually leaning too far forward. This triggers a more general upper body imbalance in which the head and chest are suspended slightly ahead of the hips and feet.

Ask a running companion to tell you if and when your head is too far forward or leaning down. The ideal position of the head is mostly upright, with your eyes focused about 30-40 yards ahead of you.

Most runners I've worked with and observed (even at the world-class level) run more efficiently and with less pain in a relatively upright body posture. There are a few runners I meet each year who have genetic spinal or other issues and naturally lean forward. In this case, each runner should do what is natural for her.

SITTING BACK

As you get tired, many runners get lazy and let the hips drop a bit. On long runs, this often results in hip soreness or pain. Avoid this by adjusting your run-walk-run early in the run to keep the muscles fresh. As you come out of a walk break, focus on being a "puppet on a string" so that all body parts are lined up, including the hips.

A BACKWARD LEAN IS RARE

It is rare for runners to lean back, but it happens. In my experience, this is usually due to a structural problem in the spine or hips. If you do this and you're having pain in the neck, back, or hips, you should see an orthopedist.

CORRECTION: "PUPPET ON A STRING"

The best correction I've found to postural problems has been this mental exercise: imagine that you are a puppet on a string. Suspended from up above like a puppet – from the head and each side of the shoulders – your head lines up with the shoulders, the hips come directly underneath, and the feet naturally touch lightly. It won't hurt anyone to do the "puppet" several times during a run.

It helps to combine this image with a deep breath. About every 4-5 minutes, as you start to run after a walk break, take a deep, lower lung breath, straighten up and say "I'm a puppet." Then imagine that you don't have to spend energy maintaining this upright posture because the strings attached from above keep you on track. As you continue to do this, you reinforce good posture as you produce a good "habit."

Upright posture not only allows you to stay relaxed, you will probably improve your stride length slightly. When you lean forward, you'll be cutting your stride to stay balanced. When you straighten up, you'll receive a stride bonus of an inch or so without any increase in energy. Note: don't try to increase stride length. If it happens by a posture improvement, it will occur naturally.

AN OXYGEN DIVIDEND

Breathing improves when you straighten up. A leaning body can't get ideal use out of the lower lungs. This can cause side pain. When you run upright, the lower lungs can receive adequate air, absorb oxygen better, and reduce the chance of side pain.

FEET LOW TO THE GROUND

The most efficient stride is a shuffle – with feet next to the ground. As long as you pick your foot up enough to avoid stumbling over a rock or uneven pavement, stay low to the ground. Most runners don't need more than one-inch clearance and can make adjustments when on uneven terrain.

Your ankle combined with the Achilles tendon will act as a spring, moving you forward on each running step. If you stay low to the ground, very little effort is required. Through this "shuffling" technique, running becomes almost automatic. When runners err on bounce, they try to push off too hard. This usually results in extra effort spent in lifting the body off the ground. You can think of this as energy wasted in the air, energy that could be used to run another mile or two.

The other negative force that penalizes those with a higher bounce is gravity. The higher you rise, the harder you will fall. Each additional bounce off the ground delivers a lot more impact on feet and legs, which on long runs produces aches, pains, and injuries.

THE CORRECTION FOR TOO MUCH BOUNCE: LIGHT TOUCH

The ideal foot placement should be so light that you don't feel yourself pushing off or landing. This means that your foot stays low to the ground and goes though an efficient and natural motion. Instead of trying to overcome gravity, you are in synch with it.

Here's a light touch drill: During the middle of a run, time yourself for 20 seconds. Focus on one item: touching so softly that you don't hear your feet. Earplugs are not allowed for this drill. Imagine that you are running on thin ice or through a bed of hot coals. Do several of these 20-second touches, becoming quieter and quieter. You should feel very little impact on your feet as you do this drill.

STRIDE LENGTH

Studies have shown that as runners get faster, the stride length shortens. This clearly shows that the key to faster and more efficient running is increased cadence or turnover of feet and legs.

A major cause of aches, pains, and injuries is a stride that is too long. Chapter 29 in this book will list aches and pains and how to correct them. But when in doubt, it is always better to err on the side of having a shorter stride.

DON'T LIFT YOUR KNEES!

Even world-class distance runners don't do this because it tires the quadriceps muscle (front of the thigh) leading to a stride that is too long to be efficient. The most common time when runners stride too long is at the end of a tiring run. This slight overstride when the legs are tired will leave your quads (front of thigh) sore the next day or two.

DON'T KICK OUT TOO FAR IN FRONT OF YOU!

If you watch the natural movement of the leg, it will kick forward slightly as the foot gently moves forward in the running motion to contact the ground. Let this be a natural motion that produces no tightness in the muscles behind the lower or upper leg.

Tightness in the front of the shin, behind the knee, or in the hamstring (back of the thigh) is a sign that you are kicking too far forward. Correct this by staying low to the ground, shortening the stride, and lightly touching the ground.

CADENCE DRILL

This easy drill improves your efficiency, making running easier. This drill excels in helping you to pull all the elements of good running form together at the same time. Over the weeks and months, if you do this drill once every week, you will find that your normal cadence slowly increases naturally.

- Warm up by walking for 5 minutes, and running and walking very gently for 10 minutes.

- Start jogging slowly for 1-2 minutes, and time yourself for 30 seconds. During this half-minute, count the number of times your left foot touches.

- Walk around for a minute or so.

- On the second 30-second drill, increase the count by 1 or 2.

- Repeat this 3-7 more times. Each time, try to increase by 1-2 additional counts.

In the process of improving turnover, the body's internal monitoring system coordinates a series of adaptations that pulls together all of the form components into an efficient team:

- Your foot touches more gently.

- Extra, inefficient motions of the foot and leg are reduced or eliminated.

- Less effort is spent on pushing up or pushing forward.

- You stay lower to the ground.

- The ankle becomes more efficient.

- Ache and pain areas are not overused.

*WA*LKING FORM

Walking form is usually not an issue when walking at a gentle, strolling pace. But every year, there are runners who get injured because they are walking in a way that aggravates some area of the foot or leg. Most of these problems come from trying to walk too fast, with too long a stride, or from using a race walking or power walking technique.

- **Avoid a long walking stride.** Maintain a relaxed motion that does not stress the knees, tendons, or muscles of the leg, feet, knees, or hips. If you feel pain or aggravation in these areas, shorten your stride. Many runners find that they can learn to walk fairly fast with a short stride. But when in doubt, use the walk for recovery and ease off.

- **Don't lead with your arms.** Minimal arm swing is best. Swinging the arms too much can encourage a longer walk stride, which can push you into aches and pains quickly. The extra rotation produced can also aggravate hip, shoulder, and neck areas. You want the legs to set the rhythm for your walk and your run. When this happens, you are more likely to get into the "zone" of the right brain.

- **Let your feet move the way that is natural for them.** When runners or walkers try techniques that supposedly increase stride length by landing farther back on the heel or pushing farther on the toe (than is natural for the individual), many get injured.

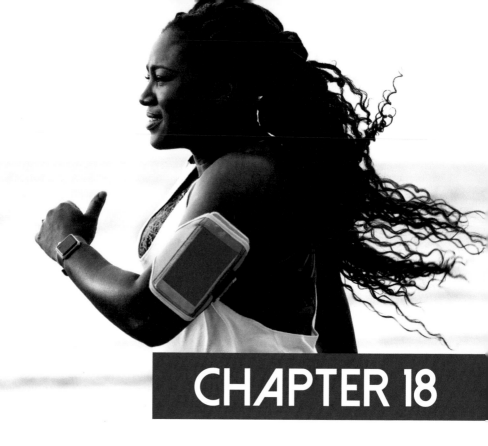

CHAPTER 18

WOMEN-SPECIFIC EXERCISE ISSUES

By Barbara Galloway

Note: For more information on these issues see *Women's Complete Guide to Running* and *Running and Fat Burning for Women*.

While most of the principles of physiology and training apply to men and women alike, there are some significant gender differences. Men tend to have larger and stronger muscles, more testosterone, and stronger bones than women. Women have wider/ flexible hips and greater fat storage. After coaching many women for over 40 years, we've found that women exercisers tend to have more patience, are more aware of the changes (especially hormonal) in their bodies, place great value in long-term health, and are more likely to back off before the aches become injuries. In this chapter, we will address the problems that only women face – with some resources.

MOVEMENT OF INTERNAL ORGANS

There is no evidence that running will cause the internal organs to move around and be damaged. Experts believe that our ancient ancestors regularly covered thousands of miles every year – probably more than most Olympic athletes today. Some who study this period of primitive human history believe that women made these constant journeys while pregnant and when carrying young children.

BREAST ISSUES

Some women are concerned that strenuous exercise can break down breast tissue. I've seen no evidence for this in any research or noted by any expert in this field. There are support and chaffing issues, which are managed daily by millions of women exercisers. Larger breasted women may have a tendency to walk or run with a slight forward lean, which can produce lower back and neck muscle fatigue and pain. The postural muscle exercises suggested in this book can help in managing this problem.

BRAS

This piece of exercise equipment is just as important as shoes for comfort and exercise enjoyment for most women. If the shoes and bra are not selected for your specific needs, you won't be very comfortable and can be miserable. You will gain a great deal of control over your comfort during exercise when you take as much time as necessary to select the model that supports you best and fits your body. Be prepared to pay significantly more than you would pay for your everyday bra. Remember that bras usually last a lot longer than shoes.

- There are a growing number of bras designed for specific types of exercise, based upon cup size. Enell, Brooks, Champion, and Nike are just a few of the brands.

- Many of the well-constructed "workout bras" are not supportive or comfortable for some women runners. The elastic in these products (for twisting and extraneous motion in tennis, pilates, etc.) allows for significant bouncing and stress when walking at a brisk pace or running.

- Comfort: Look first at the fibers next to your body. The microfibers can move moisture away from your skin. This can greatly reduce chaffing (see next section).

- A & B Cups: Women who wear these sizes can often find support with a compression bra. There will still be some movement during exercise and sometimes some skin irritation (particularly during long workouts), but this is usually minimal (see the next section on chaffing).

- C, D & E Cups: Compression bras don't work. Look for brands that have cup sizing and straps that have minimal or no elastic. Strap placement will differ among individuals so try on a variety of bras to find the configuration that matches up with your body. If you receive pressure on the shoulders where the straps press down, padded straps can help. Some large-breasted women have had success with underwire bras, especially in short runs. But on long runs, the underwire can irritate the skin.

Due to hormone fluctuations, many women find that their breasts are more sensitive at certain times of the month than others. A more supportive bra may provide more comfort when this occurs.

BRA FITTING

- Overall, the bra should fit snugly but not constrict your breathing. You want to be able to breathe naturally as the bra expands horizontally. The lower middle front of the bra should be flat across your skin – snug without pressure.

- Use the middle set of hooks when trying on the bra.

- The cup should not have wrinkles. If this is the case, try a smaller cup size. Sometimes different brands have slightly different size cups.

- If breast tissue comes out of the top of the cup or the side, try a larger size.

- The bra should not force your breasts to move in any direction, or cause them to rub together. A secure fitting cup should limit the motion.

- With the bra on, move your arms as you would do when moving the way you do during exercise. You shouldn't have any aggravation or restriction of the arm motion.

- The width is too wide if the band rides up in the back. Try lengthening the shoulder straps.

- Under the band, front and back, you should be able to insert one finger.

- Generally, you should be able to put two fingers under each strap.

- Try it on and move the way you do during exercise in front of the mirror to see if there is too much bounce.

- Run/walk in place in the dressing room or inside the store for a short distance if the store staff will let you. Ensure that you have no irritation places, that breathing is comfortable, and that you can naturally move through the range of motion you will be doing during exercise.

CHAFFING ISSUES

During warm weather and on longer workouts, most women have a few areas where clothing or body parts produce wear on other body parts. By reducing the friction in these areas, you'll reduce the irritation. The most commonly rubbed areas are between the legs, the lower front center area of the bra, and just below and behind the shoulder, where the upper arm swings behind the body. You can significantly reduce both friction and aggravation by using Vaseline and exercise products like "Glide" that tend to last longer.

Many women who have chaffing problems apply the lubricant to both skin surfaces (or the garment) before walking, and some carry a Ziplock bag with the lubricant. As in most continuous rubbing situations, the sooner you reduce the friction, the less irritation. "Compression tights" (shorts made of lycra)reduced chaffing between the legs dramatically. Sometimes, too much material or seaming in the shorts or top will increase chaffing. Minimal material is best.

INCONTINENCE

The process of childbirth, aging, and the reduction of estrogen often results in a natural weakening of support in the lower pelvis. It is fairly common that on longer walks there may be some leakage of urine. Women who experience this can do the following:

- Do kegel exercises: *visit www.mayoclinic.com/health/kegel-exercises/WOOO119*

- Carefully reduce your intake of fluids 1-2 hours before exercise or change liquids (tea is often a bladder irritant)

- Wear dark shorts and bring a change of clothing for use after exercise

- Use an absorbant pad in the shorts

- Ask your doctor about a "bladder tack"

LOSS OF MENSTRUAL PERIODS: AMENORRHEA

Years ago, a leading researcher in female fertility reported that a steady increase in weekly mileage could cause a cessation of periods. Within a few hours, he received calls from two of the leading female distance runners in the US. The first was concerned that the cessation would signify permanent loss of fertility, and he assured her that this was not indicated by the research. The second runner wanted to know if a certain amount of running was good for birth control (also not a research finding).

There are many stresses in life that can cause the interruption of the woman's monthly cycle: poor diet, low level of body fat, too much exercise, and an accumulation of life stress. When the overall stress and the stress hormone cortisol reaches a certain level in the individual, the hypothalamus in our brain reduces estrogen production and at some point menstrual periods cease or become irregular. Dr. Nicole Hagedorn, an OB/GYN, has noted that regular exercise, within your capabiliies, can reduce stress in individuals.

But when women increase their weekly distance too quickly, the increase in cortisol can be a primary cause of amenorrhea. We believe that too many miles per week kept us from conceiving for several years. It took five competitive marathons in 6 months to produce an injury, and the lack of exercise and one hormone shot during the recovery allowed for fertility to return. In other words, we owe our first child to an injury.

EXERCISING THROUGH PREGNANCY

While I ran and walked through my pregnancies, I will never say that every woman should try this. Most can probably do light exercise for the first half to two-thirds of the term. Find a doctor who wants you to exercise, if possible. When that doctor tells you not to exercise (or to cut the amount), you know that you should do so. Your doctor can be your "health coach" in the very best way. If he or she tells you not to run or exercise without any good research or reasoning, you should get a second opinion. The bottom line is that most women who are already exercising can continue for a while. Don't ever push through pain or any feeling that concerns you.

Stay cool. Exercise during the cool parts of the day. During the summer, you can alternate walking with a swim or water running (or exercise in the air conditioned indoors).

Crunch time – The final 3 months. During the last three months, the baby's demand for oxygen increases significantly. This means that it will be very easy for you to become anaerobic during workouts that were easy a month before. If your doctor is still OK with your exercise, slow down and take "sit down breaks" of 3-5 minute segments.

During this last trimester, it is very common to feel the Braxton-Hicks contractions when walking. Many doctors will tell you not to exercise when experiencing these. In my case, I was told that occasional contractions were normal and if they became stronger or more frequent, I should stop or switch exercises. I did not experience more serious contractions and continued to exercise until the day before delivery.

EXERCISING AFTER PREGNANCY

After childbirth, many women find it difficult to exercise. First, you have to recover from your childbirth experience. Coping with hormonal changes and lactation will produce fatigue also.

When you return to running after the birth of your child, assume that you are beginning all over again. Even veterans would benefit from following the beginning level program in *Women's Complete Guide to Running* or *Running: Getting Started* and adjust as needed. Start by walking gently for a few minutes every day. You will learn to treasure this time to yourself, or with a friend or two. The best exercise time of the day for me was right after nursing (or expressing milk). Walking, running, etc., is much more comfortable when you're not carrying the extra fluid and weight on your chest.

DR. DIANA TWIGGS OFFERS ADVICE AFTER RUNNING THROUGH SEVERAL PREGNANCIES

- Generally safe to continue current program of exercise, but this is not a good time to start. Gentle walking is usually OK, but check with your doctor.

- Heart rate limitations have fallen out of vogue.

- Keep your body temperature under control. This usually means less intensity, more hydration, maybe indoor exercise (with air conditioning).

- Check with your doctor concerning your limit of core temperature increase.

- Running does NOT increase miscarriage rate.

EXERCISING WHILE BREASTFEEDING

- Avoid dehydration and maintain proper nutrition to maintain milk supply.

- Long exercise sessions may slightly increase lactic acid for the next feed (not harmful but baby may not like the taste). Can always pump and dump right after if the baby doesn't like it.

- Wear properly fitting running bra for comfort.

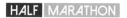

CHOOSING *A* STROLLER

- There are a number of different models. Ask several women who use them for recommendations and the cautions. The better models cost about $350 when new. Some running/walking clubs and running stores will try to match you up with women who are moving out of that phase of their life and want to sell their stroller.

- The standard wheel size is approximately 20 inches. Smaller wheels produce more bumps and don't handle uneven surface change very well.

- A safety leash is a necessity. Make sure that you have this in place and strapped securely around your arm/hand before you start. If you walk on hilly courses, a hand brake is desirable.

- Be sure that the surface and the size of the sidewalk is wide enough. **BE SAFE!**

POSTPARTUM DEPRESSION

Exercise after delivery can help women deal with the psychological challenges of childbirth. Running can help, but postpartum depression is a serious condition and needs to be treated, often with medication. See a doctor!

PMS *AND* MENSTRUAL ISSUES

Let's face it, we women are hormonally challenged. If you are experiencing significant hormonal fluctuations, see a doctor who supports exercise.

Should I exercise during my period? Most women can, and many find that they do well when the period is taking place. We're aware of at least one woman who won an Olympic gold medal during her time of the month. Planning ahead means carrying more tampons on your runs, charting a route with strategic bathrooms, wearing dark shorts, etc. Dr. Nicole Hagedorn believes that long walks may be of great benefit during the week before the period because it helps women sleep better.

Random aches, pains, and cramping are common during ovulation, before and during menses. Unusual bleeding, severe pain, etc., should be mentioned to your doctor.

Your energy level can be controlled by eating more often, combining nutrients, and moving around regularly. If you feel abnormally tired, talk to a dietitian. You may be anemic (this is common among women who have heavy periods). You should also have your hormone levels checked. Lack of sleep can be the result of low melotonin and high levels of cortosol. While unlikely, thyroid problems may be a cause. Some of the medications that women take for PMS and menstrual issues can produce fatigue and sleepiness – and other side effects. Check with your doctor or pharmacist for details.

OSTEOPOROSIS

After age 30, we lose bone mass each year. Weight-bearing exercises, such as walking and running, have been shown to strengthen the bones (or at least maintain bone density) when there is adequate calcium in the diet. Some strength exercises, such as the ones noted in this book, can also strengthen connections to the spine and help to maintain bone strength in this very important structure. Ask strength experts for other exercises that can help you. Swimming and cycling are two examples of non- weight-bearing exercises that will not promote bone density.

Technical explanation: According to Dr. John Bell, weight-bearing activities create mechanical bend forces in our bones, altering the alignment of the hydroxyapatite crystals that form bone. This causes an electrical charge of piezo electricity that stimulates the osteocyte to lay down bone.

While a moderate amount of weight-bearing exercise has been shown to stimulate bone density, doing too much (or dieting) can put exercisers into a caloric deficit. This stresses your body organism, significantly reducing estrogen production. The result is a loss of menstrual periods and reduction of bone density potential. (Reference: "The Female Athlete Triad," Running & FitNews, American Running Association, June 1999.) When you add the stress of pounding types of exercise (high impact aerobics, fast running, etc.), stress fracture risk increases rapidly according to our experience. You can reduce this risk by exercising longer one day and resting from running the next day. It also helps on long walks to insert liberal shuffle breaks from the beginning.

PREVENTION

Exercise can help young women, in effect, put bone density "into storage." About 90% of female bone strength is established by the age of 18, and density peaks between age 25 and 30.

Those who exercise strenuously and consume adequate calcium have a higher level of peak bone density. "Think of bone mass as a bank account that needs to be filled with the help of calcium and exercise to ensure strong bones later." Catherine Niewochner, MD.

"Although calcium intake is often cited as the most important factor in healthy bones, our study suggests that exercise is really the predominant lifestyle determinant of bone strength in young women." Professor Tom Lloyd, Pennsylvania State College of Medicine. (References: *Journal of Applied Physiology*, Oct 2004 and *Journal of Pediatrics*, June 2004.)

After the age of 30, bone density tends to decrease with each passing year. The object is to start with the highest level possible and then hold on to what you have. Weight-bearing exercise (60 minutes every other day) and calcium intake (especially milk products and dark green vegetables) are two of the best activities to accomplish this. Most can also do a short walk on the alternate day. The US National Institute of Health recommends that those above the age of 10 years old consume at least 1000mg of calcium a day (approximately three 8oz yogurts).

At menopause, the recommendation rises to a minimum daily dose of 1500mg (diet plus supplements). Vitamin D is crucial for calcium absorption: 400IU is recommended for adults. As always, consult with your doctor about any individual issues or medical problems.

BONE LOSS RISK BEHAVIORS

- Smoking: if you smoke, or are around second-hand smoke, try to quit and avoid a smoky environment.
- Too much alcohol: no more than 2 glasses of wine or 2 beers per day.
- Too much caffeine: limit to 3 cups of coffee per day or equivalent.
- Simple carbohydrate consumption: sugar, refined flour, sports drinks instead of milk. Limit simple carb consumption to no more than 20% of total carbohydrate consumption per day.
- Salt: if you need to add to the taste of food, add a little and avoid regular ingestion of salty foods.
- Laxative use – try to limit to occasional use if needed.
- Restrictive and prolonged diets: diets don't tend to achieve long-term fat loss anyway.
- Cortisone drugs – consult with your doctor about drug issues.

MENOPAUSE AND AFTER

All post-menopausal women should consider supplemental calcium and vitamin D (especially if sun exposure is limited) in order to prevent osteoporosis. There are a continuing series of questions about hormone replacement (estrogen). Read about the options and discuss with your doctor. While estrogen promotes calcium absorption and a reduction of cardiovascular disease, it may increase risk of breast cancer, blood clots, and endometrial cancer.

Research shows that exercise continues to enhance bone density past the age of 50. Studies of middle aged and post-menopausal women have found that, at least every other day exercise, adding up to more than 7 miles total a week resulted in increased bone density in the trunk. Walking and running also produced a density increase in the femoral neck bones.

Bone density tests can usually tell you whether you're at risk for osteoporosis. Dr. Richard S. Newman, from the American Medical Athletic Association and ARA website, recommends that those possibly at risk for osteoporosis, should talk to their doctors about a "DEXA scan."

This sonogram technology calculates bone density in a 15-minute session, fully clothed on an exam table. There are other tests, including a CT scan test. Osteoporosis is indicated when your bone density reading shows that you are a certain percentage below peak density, based on age.

Exercise, calcium, and vitamin D supplementation and medication can help you hold the bone density you have. There are also some drugs that have been very effective in this area (Fosamax for example). Again, talk to your doctor.

MENOPAUSE

Most exercising women who are going through menopause tell me that they feel better and have a better attitude on the walking/running days. Exercise helps women sleep better, combating the insomnia that is common.

The symptoms and intensity of menopause differ greatly. Your greatest asset is a doctor who understands the benefits/effects of exercise and wants you to do it. After you talk through most of the symptoms and make some minor adjustments, you will find what works for you. But whenever you have a possible medical issue, run it by your doctor.

Your energy level can be controlled by eating more often, combining nutrients, and moving around regularly. If you feel abnormally tired, talk to a dietician. Thyroid problems are common as we age, and significant loss of energy can be a symptom. If you've tried to deal with your energy loss through nutrition, etc., without success, ask your doctor about possible thyroid issues. You should have your hormone levels checked. Lack of sleep can be the result of low melotonin and high levels of cortosol.Hormone supplementation is a very complex issue and should be discussed with your doctor. Because of the reduction of estrogen production, during and after menopause, and sleeplessness due to low melotonin, many women respond well to supplements. OB/GYN Nicole Hagedorn believes that when supplementation is advised, "bioidentical hormones" work better for most women. These have the same molecular structure as the ones produced by your body. As with all important medical issues, check with your doctor.

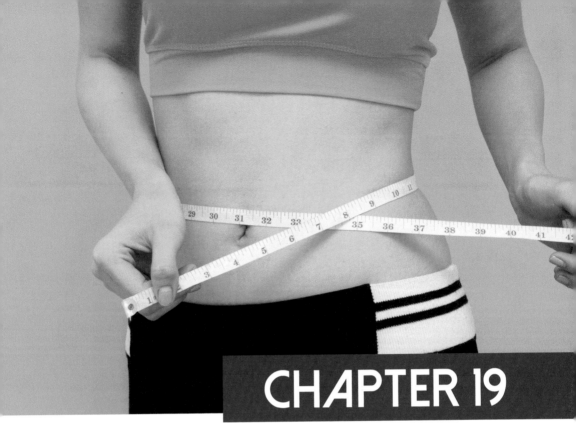

CHAPTER 19

HOW TO BURN FAT DURING
A HALF MARATHON TRAINING PROGRAM

Many women want to use their increase in half marathon training to burn off some fat, which will improve times in long races and improve health. If you stay focused and use the right tools, it is possible to have a sustainable fat loss during a half marathon training program. But if you don't monitor nutrients and intake, you may deprive yourself of the protein, calcium, iron, etc., that you need for repair. But first, let's destroy some myths.

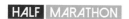

HALF MARATHON EATING MYTHS

I'll lose a lot of weight when training for a half marathon.

In fact, losing a lot of weight the wrong way can leave you weak, without the energy or essential nutrients needed for endurance performance. Too much of a calorie deficit can produce a blood sugar level inadequate for finishing a run – or even starting one.

You can eat anything desired when training for a half marathon.

This myth is more of an excuse that runners give themselves for "gratification eating." Because they finished a 12-mile training run, some runners give themselves permission to eat a box of Girl Scout cookies or to eat big meals for 3 days afterward. Don't go there!

HALF MARATHON GOAL CAN BE A CATALYST

At every big event expo, I talk to at least a dozen women who tell me that they lost 30-100 pounds or more because they set the goal of finishing a half marathon. In some cases it took 10 years, but as I talked with each, there were two concepts that were shared and followed:

1. They set up a cognitive plan to monitor eating. This empowers the conscious brain to choose and account for food consumed. This frontal lobe brain component overrides the subconscious brain, which can stimulate subconscious "gratification snacks." (Suddenly you realize that the potato chip bag is empty and you are the only one who has been eating them.)

2. They used one of my training books and kept up with the training schedule. Exercise does a lot more than just burn calories. When you run or walk, for more than about 30 minutes, you activate circuits in the brain that burn fat, control appetite, and make you feel good about what you are doing. This reduces the chance that the subconscious brain will trigger "gratification eating" to combat the "blues."

THE RULES

1. Reload your muscle fuel within 30 minutes of finishing a run.

2. Set a realistic calorie deficit – between 50 and 300 calories per day.

3. Write down everything you eat.

4. Track your food intake and exercise with an app or a website.

5. Each day, see if you are getting your nutrients: vitamins, minerals, protein.

6. Get a step counter and strive to take 10,000 steps or more per day.

7. Run/walk for a minimum of 60 minutes on the two maintenance days and 90 minutes on the non-long run weekend.

8. Ensure that your blood sugar level is adequate during the half hour before a workout or race and during long workouts/races.

TAKE THESE STEPS TO *A* "LIGHTER YOU"

1. **Eat a "reloading snack" within 30 minutes of finishing a run.**
   There are circuits in the brain that are triggered to reload the fuel you burned during the first 30 minutes of your run. If you don't reload within 30 minutes of finishing, you will not have the energy supplies you need during the first part of your next run. Many runners tell me that avoiding the reloading meal leaves them hungrier later. The best mix of reloading nutrients, according to research, is 80% simple carbohydrates and 20% protein. The products Accelerade and Endurox R4 have this in the mix. The brain's hunger/satisfaction circuit is more likely to be on the satisfaction side if you have consumed your snack within the half hour of completion. In this meal, avoid fat, dairy products, and foods with fiber.

GUIDELINES FOR RELOADING

- 4 miles or less – 100 calories

- 4-8 miles – 150 calories

- 8-12 miles – 200 calories

- 12-16 miles – 250 calories

- 16+ miles – 300 calories

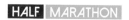

2. **Set a realistic calorie deficit – between 50 and 300 calories per day.**
By focusing on a congnitive strategy, you engage the frontal lobe and assume conscious control over eating behaviors. A deficit of 50-300 calories per day can be sustainable, whereas higher deficits are likely to engage the "starvation circuit" in your brain. While you are depriving yourself of the amount that the starvation circuit feels is adequate, the circuit remembers. When you resume eating regularly, it triggers a hunger response and overeating. This is one reason why starvation diets don't work and result in more fat deposited (than was lost) during the year after the diet is terminated.

3. **Get a step counter and strive to take 10,000 steps or more per day.**
Walking steps, taken in amounts of 100 to 1,000 increments, burn fat, increase your "calorie budget" for the day, and don't tend to trigger the hunger circuit. Many runners find that increasing walking steps creates most or all of the calorie deficit they need, requiring little or no change in food intake to produce the calorie burn desired.

4. **Write down everything you eat.**
This is the most powerful tool to control food intake. The act of writing, by itself, activates the conscious brain triggering circuits monitor food intake, avoid "decadent" food, and stay away from subconscious gratification eating.

5. **Each day, do an accounting of your nutrients.**
Use the app or website of your choice (such as www.myfitnesspal.com or www.fitday.com) and see if your diet gave you the vitamins, minerals, protein, etc., needed. This conscious brain exercise will allow you to search for and prepare foods that fill in the deficits. You'll also receive your calorie balance for the day. By mentally focusing on this at least once a day, you'll tend to make executive decisions about what to eat instead of slipping into subconscious gratification eating patterns. There are many free websites that have tools to help you in your calorie accounting, charting progress, search for foods, etc.

6. **Run/walk for a minimum of 60 minutes on the two maintenance days and 90 minutes on the non-long-run weekend.**
Avoid huffing and puffing and choose a gentle pace. Fast running burns glycogen but not fat. Use the Run-Walk-Run strategy that works best for you, but don't be shy about using more walk breaks if you are huffing and puffing or are not feeling as good as usual – especially during the first 15 minutes of the run. The fat-burning circuits don't reach their maximum capacity until about 40 minutes into the run – only if you are exercising at a comfortable level of exertion (avoiding huffing and puffing). Continuing to run at that point extends and maintains fat-

burning adaptations. If you're not running 60 or 90 minutes now, gradually work up to that level.

7. **Ensure that your blood sugar level (BSL) is adequate during the half hour before a workout or race.**

When you're in a calorie deficit, you're more likely to have a drop in the BSL at various times of the day – especially in the afternoon. By eating a blood sugar booster snack you will tend to feel more motivated and feel better during the run. On early morning runs, the BSL is usually adequate. If the snack is mostly sugar, you should consume it within 30 minutes before the start of your run, with a small glass of water.

8. **Don't radically change diet when training for a challenging goal.**

Every year, I hear from several dozen women who have to abandon a training program because of dietary issues. They started or restarted their running career and made a radical change in their diets at the same time. After several weeks or months they either felt chronically fatigued or experienced some digestive issues. A more successful strategy is to make small and gradual changes, while monitoring nutrition by a website, such as *www.fitday.com*. Note: The section Nutrition for Runners has more information in this area.

Note: You'll find much more information on this topic, including BSL snacks, recipes, etc., in our book *Running and Fat Burning for Women*, from www.RunInjuryFree.com. Following is an example of Barbara's tips that you can present to your conscious brain to keep you on a healthy eating track.

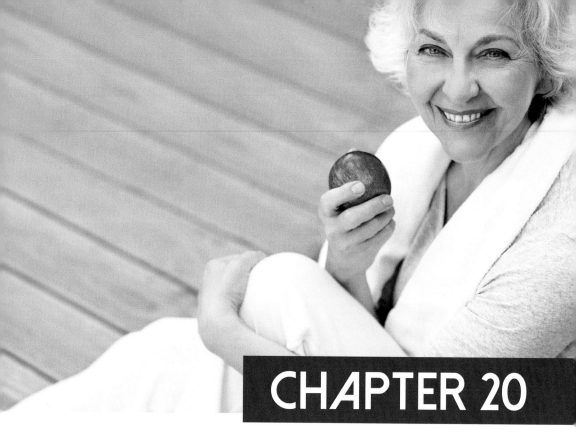

CHAPTER 20

EATING WITH A PURPOSE

Conscious brain control over eating by Barbara Galloway

- Eat mostly at home; you don't have control over what is included in restaurant food.

- At the grocery store, fill up the cart first in the produce section. Choose a variety of colorful vegetables and some fruits, nuts, and seeds.

- Know the calorie content and nutrient breakdown of what you're eating (read the label or use a website like *www.fitday.com*).

- Concentrate on the positive: "I can eat more of (good tasting fruit and crunchy vegetables") rather than "I have to eat less of _____".

- Visualize the food on your plate as being in your stomach. Ask yourself "Do I want to stretch my stomach to cram in more food" "Do I need that much right now?"

- Don't have more than 3 items or "dishes" at one meal.

- Drink a glass of water (6-8oz) before eating, and drink 4-6 oz during the meal.

- Hot fluids (tea, coffee, broth) leave you feeling fuller than cold fluids.

- If you are very hungry, never eat fatty appetizers before a meal. Instead, choose soup, salad, hot tea, warm skim milk.

- Take vitamins with a meal and avoid caffeine for half an hour.

- Don't even think about going to a buffet.

- Visit the grocery store with a mission. Have a list of exactly what you will buy and only buy what is on the list.

- Veggies: steam, toast, or stir-fry – or eat them raw or in salads.

- Use non-fat dressings or spray-on dressings for salads.

- Eat slowly! Increase the number of chews for each bite – this triggers more satisfaction in the stomach.

- Count every calorie eaten – it only hurts you to "forget" the amount or certain foods in your totals.

- Fluid calories add up quickly. Budget your alcohol, fruit juice, etc.

- Buy the highest quality foods: lean meats, fruits, veggies, and whole grain products. These may cost a little more but you'll appreciate the quality, especially when the taste is better. You will feel better about the quality of your nutrition.

- Herbs and spices can enhance the savory flavor of foods, leaving you satisfied with fewer calories consumed.

- Try to accumulate your daily quota of vitamins and minerals from food. If your daily analysis of nutrients shows regular deficiencies (based on the recommended daily allowance, RDA) then find a really good vitamin. Jeff travels a lot and takes Cooper Complete vitamins, designed by Dr. Kenneth Cooper.

- In choosing a restaurant, check out the websites to find one that breaks down the nutritional composition of the menu items. By planning ahead, you can avoid impulsive gratification eating.

- Another option is to get a nutritional guide when you arrive at the restaurant and analyze it before the waiter takes your order.

- Try to avoid or severely limit trans fat and saturated fat. Use olive oil or eat fish that have omega-3 oil.

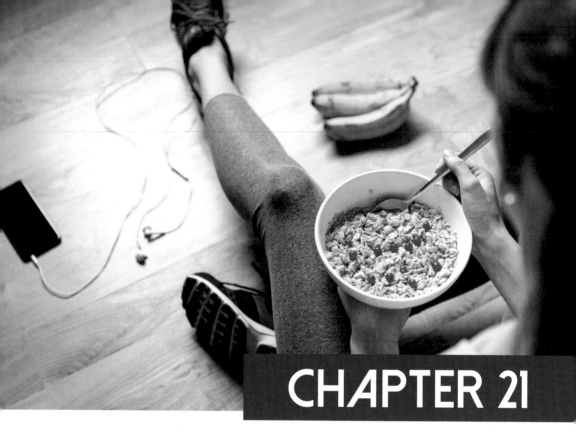

CHAPTER 21

AN EXERCISER'S DIET

As an endurance athlete, you will not need a significant increase in vitamins and minerals, protein, etc. But if you don't get these ingredients for several days in a row, you will feel less energized and more tired. By following the guidelines below and monitoring nutrition by an app or website, you can avoid "running out of gas."

MOST IMPORTANT NUTRIENT: *WATER*

Whether you prefer water, juice, or other fluids, drink regularly throughout the day. Strive for 8 x 8 oz (240ml) glasses. Caffeine drinks only deliver half of the fluid for absorption. Alcohol has a dehydrating effect.

If you have to take bathroom stops during walks or runs, you are drinking too much – either before or during the exercise. During an exercise session of 60 minutes or less, most exercisers don't need to drink at all. The intake of fluid before exercise should be arranged so that the excess fluid is eliminated before the run. Each person is a bit different, so you will have to find a routine that works for you.

SWEAT THE ELECTROLYTES

Electrolytes are the salts that your body loses when you sweat: sodium, potassium, magnesium, and calcium. When these minerals get too low, your fluid transfer system doesn't work as well and you may experience ineffective cooling, swelling of the hands, and other problems. Most runners have no problem replacing these in a normal diet, but if you are regularly experiencing cramping during or after exercise, you may be low in sodium or potassium. The best product I've found for replacing these minerals is called SUCCEED. If you have high blood pressure (or any issue with electrolytes), get your doctor's guidance before taking any salt supplement.

PRACTICAL EATING ISSUES

- Most runners don't need to eat before a run unless blood sugar is low. In that case, consume 100 calories of a blood sugar booster you have successfully used before.

- Reload most effectively by eating within 30 min of the finish of a run (80% carb/20% rotein).

- During long runs and races the rule of thumb is 2-4 oz of water, every 2 miles.

- Blood sugar booster rule of thumb during long runs and races: 30-40 calories every 2 miles. Use various snacks during long runs to find the one that works best for you: gummi bears, hard candy, gels, energy bars, sugar cubes, etc.

- Eating or drinking too much right before the start of a run can interfere with lower lung breathing and may cause side pain. The food or fluid in your stomach limits your intake of air into the lower lungs and restricts the action of the diaphragm.

- If you are running low on blood sugar at the end of your long runs, increase your blood sugar booster snacks from the beginning of your next run (see the next chapter for more information).

- It is never a good idea to eat a huge meal – especially the night before a long run or a race. Those who claim that they must "carbo load" with a large meal the night before are rationalizing their desire to eat a lot of food. Eating a big meal the night before (or the day of) a long run can result in "unloading" during the run.

When you are sweating a lot, it is a good idea to drink several glasses a day of a good electrolyte beverage (not when running). Accelerade, by Pacific Health Labs, is the best I've seen for both maintaining fluid levels and electrolyte levels.

RUN

- As soon as you awaken, drink either a cup of coffee or a glass of water.

- 30 min before any run (if blood sugar is low): approx. 100 calories of a blood sugar booster snack.

- Within 30 min after a run: approx. 200 calories of an 80% carb/20% protein (Endurox R4, for example).

- If you are sweating a lot during hot weather, 2-3 glasses of a good electrolyte beverage like Accelerade throughout the day plus your normal intake of water (6-8 glasses recommended).

Hint: Caffeine, when consumed before exercise, engages the systems that enhance running and extend endurance, but only half of the fluid will be absorbed.

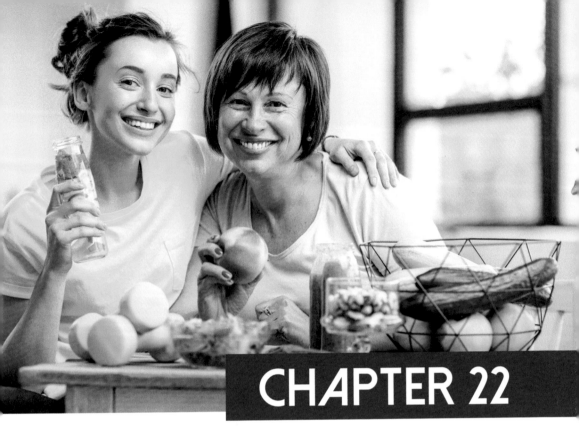

CHAPTER 22

GOOD BLOOD SUGAR = MOTIVATION

Your brain is fueled by blood sugar. When the blood sugar level (BSL) is at a good, moderate "normal" level, you feel good, stable, and motivated. But if the BSL is lowered or interrupted, the brain starts shutting things down.

If you eat too much sugar, 45 or more minutes before you run, your BSL can rise too high. You'll feel really good for a short period, but the excess sugar triggers a release of insulin. This reduces BSL to an uncomfortable level. In this state, your energy drops, mental focus is foggy, and motivation goes down rapidly.

When blood sugar level is maintained throughout the day, you will be more motivated to exercise, add other movement to your life, be mentally active, deal with stress, and solve problems. Just as eating throughout the day keeps metabolism up, the steady infusion of balanced nutrients all day long will maintain stable BSL. This produces a feeling of well-being.

You don't want to get on the "bad side" of your BSL. Low levels are a stress on the brain – literally messing with your mind. If you have not eaten for several hours before a run-walk, you'll receive an increase in the number of negative and anxiety hormones reducing motivation to exercise.

The simple act of eating about 100 calories of 80% simple carbohydrate and about 20% protein within 30 minutes before running can reduce the negative, make you feel good, and get you out the door. This can be the difference in getting out to run – or not.

THE BSL ROLLER COASTER

Eating a snack with too many calories of simple carbohydrate can be counterproductive for BSL maintenance. As mentioned, when the sugar level gets too high, your body produces insulin, sending BSL lower than before. The tendency is to eat again, which produces excess calories that are converted into fat. But if you don't eat, you'll stay hungry and pretty miserable – in no mood to exercise, to move around and burn calories, or get in your run for the day.

TRY EATING EVERY 2-3 HOURS

Once it is established which snacks work best to maintain your BSL, most people maintain a stable blood sugar level by eating small meals regularly, every 2-3 hours. As noted in the previous chapter, it's best to combine complex carbs with protein and a small amount of fat.

DO I HAVE TO EAT BEFORE RUNNING?

Only if your blood sugar is low. Most who run-walk in the morning, don't need to eat anything before the start. As mentioned, if your blood sugar level is low in the afternoon, and you have a run scheduled, a snack can help when taken about 30 minutes before the run. If you feel that a morning snack will help, the only issue is to avoid consuming so much that you get an upset stomach.

For best results in raising blood sugar when it is too low (within 30 minutes before a run), a snack should have about 80% of the calories in simple carbohydrate and 20% in protein. This promotes the production of insulin, which is helpful before a run in getting the glycogen into your muscles and ready for use. The product Accelerade has worked best among the thousands of runners I hear from every year. It has the 80%/20% ratio of carb to protein. If you eat an energy bar with the 80/20 ratio, be sure to drink 4-6 oz of water with it.

EATING DURING EXERCISE

Most exercisers don't need to worry about eating or drinking during a run until the length exceeds 90 minutes. At this point, there are several options. In this case, most runners wait until the 30-40 minute mark in the workout before starting to take the blood sugar level (BSL) booster. Diabetics may need to eat sooner and more often, but this is an individual issue.

The brain's fuel is blood glucose. If you don't keep this boosted during a long run, the brain will be deprived and will start shutting things down. Avoid this by trying different snacks and using the one that works best for you.

Rule of thumb: 30-40 calories about every 2 miles (20-25 minutes) with 2-4 oz of water (60-120 ml).

GU or gel products – these come in small packets and are the consistency of honey or thick syrup. The most successful way to take them is to put 1-3 packets in a small plastic bottle with a pop-top. About every 10-15 minutes, take a small amount with a sip or two of water. These products have caused nausea more often than simple sugar products, so try them out many times before using in a race.

Energy bars – Cut into small pieces. Avoid products with a lot of fiber, fat, or protein.

Candy – Particularly gummi bears or hard candies, such as Lifesavers.

Sugar cubes or tablets – This is the simplest of the BSL booster snacks and the easiest on the stomach for most runners.

Sports drinks – I've noticed that a significant percentage of my runners who drink sports drinks during a run experience nausea, so this is not my top recommendation. If you have found this to work for you, use it exactly as you have used it before. A sports drink like Accelerade is helpful the day before or after a strenuous run. During a run, I recommend water.

IT IS IMPORTANT TO RELOAD AFTER EXERCISE – WITHIN 30 MINUTES

Whenever you have finished a hard or long workout (for you), a recovery snack can help you recover faster. Again, the 80/20 ratio of simple carbohydrate to protein has been most successful in reloading the muscles. The product that has worked best among the thousands I work with each year is Endurox R4.

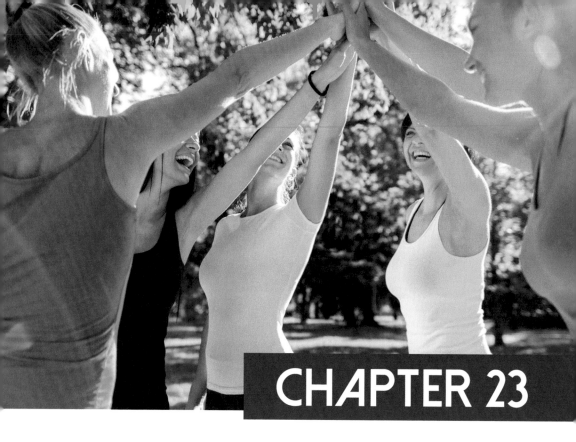

CHAPTER 23

YOUR MOTIVATION TRAINING PLAN

We are surrounded by a sea of stress. If we go with the flow of how we feel, we'll allow the subconscious brain to secrete anxiety and negative attitude hormones, which will send our attitude rising and falling like the tide. Your mission is to have strategies in place to shift control into the executive brain in the frontal lobe for smooth and confident sailing.

By developing and using cognitive strategies, you can train your mind to move from one thought to the next – just as you train your body to go one more mile or one more walk break. This manages the flow of negative hormones and turns on circuits to move you forward, step by step.

Most of the day, most of the routine activities are monitored and managed by the subconscious, reflex brain. One of its functions is to monitor stress and start shutting things down (like motivation) when the stress level is too high. Having a plan in advance that you believe in will help you shift brain control into the frontal lobe – the conscious brain. Focusing on one small (and doable) step at a time reduces stress significantly and allows the frontal lobe to override the negativity of the reflex brain. By moving from one step to the next, you maintain conscious control over your motivation and training, reprograming the subconscious brain to get moving, get out the door, keep going, break through barriers, and be strong to the finish. As you practice and fine tune these cognitive strategies, the process becomes easier and easier. Here are the major concepts:

- Do a reality check on your goal. Make sure that it is within your current capabilities and that you have enough time to perform the key workouts while resting between. Keep evaluating your goals and adjust as you head toward the key dates on your calendar. This maintains conscious control over the process.

- Acknowledge that the subconscious brain responds to stress by sending negative hormone messages to lower motivation. Under severe stress, this reflex brain will reduce blood flow to the gut, frontal lobe, and damaged areas to create pain. Start talking to the reflex brain when this starts to happen, laugh, and tell it to open up the blood flow. This shifts brain activity into the executive brain where you can take conscious control.

- Diffuse the stress by using one or more of the simple methods listed below or one that you design. Keep telling the reflex brain that you know what it is doing and that you will not let this happen.

- Move forward by walking. Even if you are not going to run immediately, walk around the room thinking through the next steps in the "Jump Start" program. Use the mantras that help you shift gears. The conscious shift to positive thoughts can change the mood in a few minutes by triggering the release of positive peptides.

- When it is time for your run, go through the "Jump Start" program in the book *Mental Training for Runners*. As you run/walk/run, the endorphins you release will lock into receiver sites all over the body, transmitting messages that you feel good, you can do it.

- During the run, or during other quiet periods (driving in a car, waiting for a flight or a meeting, etc.), identify the challenges you want to manage or overcome. List the negative messages you receive and the problems in past experiences. Then rehearse yourself through each situation.

- Concentrate on one challenge at a time. As you fine tune your strategy, you will get better at moving quickly to positive action.

- Break up the challenge into a series of small steps that take you from the beginning of the challenge to the successful finish.

- Mentally rehearse the steps during various quiet periods of your day. Even if you don't know the solution to problems that come up, rehearse yourself digging down, getting through it, and finishing with a great feeling of accomplishment.

- As you repeat the rehearsal and fine tune it, you are re-programming the reflex brain to automatically move from one step to the next when confronted with the challenge.

As long as you have the challenge, continue the regular rehearsal – adjusting to your situation, making it better and better.

Note: For more information on this topic with step-by-step instructions, see our book *Mental Training for Runners*, available autographed at www.JeffGalloway.com.

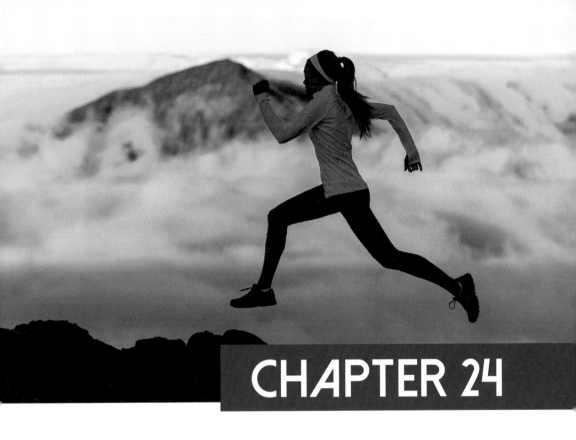

CHAPTER 24

MENTAL TRAINING PROGRAMS

By using cognitive strategies, you gain control over your motivation while reducing fatigue and injury risk.

- Training programs can re-program the subconscious reflex brain.
- You have the power to take charge over motivation and improve attitude.
- Rehearsal drills – break up a task into doable steps, performed step by step.
- Magic words tap into successful patterns and our intuitive/creative powers.
- Dirty tricks will distract your reflex brain – activate the frontal lobe.
- How to manage/eliminate pain's hold over your motivation.

The choice is yours. You can take control over your attitude, or you can let your reflex brain go through a series of negative reactions that usually result in low motivation and reduced performance. By using the proven strategies in this chapter you can turn a negative attitude into a positive one, reprogram the reflex brain to stay on track to a positive goal, and tap into the incredible powers of the conscious right brain. Whether you struggle to get out the door when running by yourself, or you need more motivation to keep going when it's tough, you have a better chance of success when you have a strategy. This is your motivational training program.

To understand motivation, look inside the mental command and response center. The center of action, especially when under physical challenges, is the subconscious reflex brain. When stress accumulates to a significant level, this powerful center takes protective action to reduce motivation and reduce effort level.

A stream of messages is released telling us to "slow down," "stop and you'll feel better," "this isn't your day," and even philosophical messages like, "why are you doing this." Stress secretions of peptides lock into sites all over the body transmitting an emotional environment that is unmotivated and negative. The reflex brain also reduces blood flow to areas of damage that it has already identified. This results in a sensation of pain that normally would not be felt based upon the damage itself, a condition called TMS (Tension Myositis Syndrome).

Note: I am not suggesting that you should run through pain when there is chance of a serious injury. When you have pain in a weak link area that you suspect is an injury, check with your doctor to verify. In many cases, the pain is stress-induced TMS and can be managed. (See my *Mental Training for Runners* book for more about TMS.)

By engaging the conscious brain in the frontal lobe, we can stay on track and possibly push to a higher level of performance, even when there is significant stress. The series of mental training drills in this chapter have been very successful in re-programming the reflex brain. With the conscious brain in charge, you can back off the effort if there is a legitimate issue of health or safety (very rare), or check your "Magic Mile" to ensure that your goal is not out of your current range of ability.

These drills can allow you to move from one doable step to the next. By managing pace and diffusing stress, the creative and intuitive right side of the frontal lobe can be active and search for solutions to current problems, with connections to your inner resources, engaging the spirit.

DRILL 1 - REHEARSING SUCCESS

Rehearsal has been used for decades by individuals in various fields to achieve their potential on any given day, under a variety of conditions. Mentally envisioning a series of challenges and rewards, all the way to the goal, gears up the mind/body team to work together at top capacity.

- Rehearsing realistic fatigue, aches, and pains, negative messages, doubts, etc., desensitizes one to the challenges.

- A series of small steps. The conscious frontal lobe reprograms the reflex brain to stay focused by breaking down a challenge into segments, one leading automatically to the next to the successful finish.

- As the rehearsal is repeated and fine tuned, the reflex brain can be reprogrammed to move you from one positive step to the next instead of responding to the negative motivation reflex due to stress/pressure.

Rehearsal drills are listed in the "Situations" chapter of our book *Mental Training for Runners*, with step-by-step formats. The principles are as follows:

What: This is a mental storyline of how you want the experience to unfold. At first, you may focus on specific parts of a workout or a race that has been challenging for you. You may continue to rehearse only the challenging parts or tie the parts into a continuous preview of the whole experience.

Most runners "fast forward" through the less challenging segments and focus on the "issues" that have caused problems. An experienced rehearser can move though a marathon rehearsal within a matter of 2-3 minutes at the end of a season.

When: Rehearsals can be done during a run, when driving, in the shower, waiting for a flight, etc. Trying out the rehearsal during a hard workout can help you fine tune it to be more effective. Many go through key rehearsal segments during long runs.

Be realistic and positive: The effectiveness of this mental drill will depend upon how complete and honest you were about the real challenges, how often and effective you rehearsed, how open you are to make adjustments, dig down as you get through the struggle. It's also important to visualize finishing with pride, satisfaction, and a great sense of accomplishment.

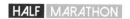

Desensitize: Revisit the negative messages that have been experienced during challenging workouts or races and every significant physical challenge that could happen during the event. As you rehearse getting through these, you desensitize yourself to surprises that could add stress during the event.

Rehearse the problem, even if you don't know the solution: By envisioning a past problem that you haven't solved, including your "digging down" and getting through it, you empower the creative/intuitive right brain to find solutions. It often does this by race day (often without sending a message).

A series of small steps: Challenges are not confronted head on, but segmented into doable units. So when there is a significant hill that you are worried about, visualize shortening the run segments, shortening stride length, accomplishing one segment at a time, and not focusing on the top of the hill until you are congratulating yourself for moving over the top, smoothly gliding down the other side.

Each segment leads automatically to the next: By rehearsing the segments attached to one another, you are more likely to move from one to the next when you get into the challenge.

Rehearse a variety of weather conditions, aches, and pains, etc.: As you envision a variety of possible challenges, you will be better prepared for what could happen. You are training the various body/mind components to work as a team to get the job done while making adjustments for the conditions of the day.

Finish with a vision of success/accomplishment: Always rehearse success that is realistic. Yes, you feel tired, but you crossed the finish with strength and dignity. Focusing too specifically on a goal that is too ambitious can disconnect the brain circuits that could help you with doable performances.

DRILL 2 - MAGIC WORDS

Even the most motivated person has periods during a tough workout or race when he or she wants to abandon the goal. By using a successful brainwashing technique, you can use the resources from past successes to pull you through these negative thoughts and feel like a champion at the end. Associate these successes with key words, and you can build on this success and confidence with each use.

Think back to the common and significant problems that you face in your tough workouts or races. These are the ones that are most likely to challenge you again. As you go through a series of speed sessions and long runs, you will confront just about every problem you will face. Go back in your memory bank and pull out instances when you started to lose motivation due to these but finished and overcame the challenge.

My Three Magic Words: Relax ... Power ... Glide

In really tough runs, I have three challenges that occur over and over:

1. I become tense when I get really tired, worried that I will struggle badly at the end.

2. I feel the loss of the bounce and strength I had at the beginning, and worry that there will be no strength later.

3. My form starts to get ragged, and I worry about further deterioration of muscles and tendons and more fatigue due to "wobbling."

The problems themselves are almost never serious. The key word is "worry." When you focus on the negative possibilities, you stimulate negative hormones and build anxiety. This adds stress to the reflex brain, which will trigger more negative attitude peptides. So by focusing on problems and predicting negative outcomes, you will lose motivation and realize what you are projecting.

My big motivational breakthrough was learning to counter these three problems with the magic words "Relax ... Power ... Glide." The visualization of each of these positives shifts mental control to the conscious frontal lobe of the brain. The real magic comes from the association I have made with hundreds of successful experiences when I started to "lose it" in one of the three areas but overcame the problems. Each time I "run through" one or more of the challenges, I associate the experience with these magic words and add to the magic. Positive peptides are released, attitude improves, stress is released, and confidence returns.

Now, when something starts to go wrong, I repeat the three words, over and over. Instead of increasing my anxiety, the repetition of the words calms me down (negative hormones are neutralized) and shifts me into my conscious brain. Even though I don't feel as strong in the last mile as I did in the first one, I'm empowered just by knowing that I have a strategy and can draw upon my past experience (more positive attitude hormones are secreted).

And when my legs lose the efficient path and bounce, the right frontal lobe is empowered to take over and make adjustments, finding inner strength to go on, as it has in past successes.

When I say magic words that are associated with successful experience, there are two positive effects. The saying of the words floods the brain with positive memories. For a while, the negative messages of the left brain don't have a chance and you can get down the course for a half mile or more. But the second effect may be more powerful. The words directly link you to the right brain, which works intuitively to make the same connections that allowed you to solve the problems before.

To be successful on any day, you must first finish the race. Most of the time, you can get through the "bad parts" by not giving up, and simply putting one foot in front of the other. As you push beyond the negative left brain messages, you create the confidence to do this again and again. Each time you use the magic words and feel the results, you are reprogramming the reflex brain. Feel free to use my magic words or develop your own. The more experiences you have associated with the words, the more magic.

DRILL 3 - PLAYING DIRTY TRICKS ON THE REFLEX BRAIN

The strategy of the rehearsal drill will get you focused and organized while reducing the stress for at least the first third of the race or workout. Magic words can pull you along through most of the remaining challenging sessions. But on the really rough days, it helps to have some dirty tricks to play on the reflex brain.

These are quick fixes that distract the reflex brain's "garbage" messages for a while, allowing you to keep going for the next segment of the course. These imaginative and sometimes crazy images don't have to have any logic behind them.

But when you counter a reflex brain anxiety with a creative idea, you shift control into the frontal lobe, activating the creative right side. The flow of negative messages stops for a while.

The conscious action and the image of each trick, as mentioned next, will shift action to the executive brain where you can take command. This can change the peptides from negative to positive. Having fun with these visualizations will unlock more positive hormones, improving confidence and attitude.

A shift to creative images can further shift action to the right brain of your frontal lobe. This often triggers a series of creative thoughts that can entertain you. Once engaged, the right brain can subconsciously solve problems, boost your inner resolve to keep going, find hidden strength, etc.

DIRTY TRICK: THE GIANT INVISIBLE RUBBER BAND

When I get tired at the end of a hard race, I unpack this secret weapon and throw it around someone ahead of me – or someone who had the audacity to pass me. For a while, the person doesn't realize that he or she has been "looped" and continues to push onward while I get the benefit of being pulled along. After a minute or two of mentally projecting myself into this image, I have to laugh for believing in such an absurd notion. When you take charge over the situation by projecting a set of behaviors and acting on them, you activate the conscious brain to take control. Furthermore, laughing activates the creative/resourceful right side. This usually generates several more entertaining ideas, especially when you do this on a regular basis.

The right brain has millions of dirty and entertaining tricks. Once you get it rolling, you're likely to receive intuitive solutions to current problems. It can stimulate new thoughts as you get closer to your finish, step by step. Most importantly, this circuit can empower the legs, feet, and muscles to do what they are capable of doing on that day. The result will often surprise you.

MORE DIRTY TRICKS:

- **The jet engine behind you**
  When you start to slow down, imagine that there is a jet engine from a giant 777 aircraft that is blasting you from behind – run in this tailwind.

- **Oxygen molecules in your shirt**
  When you are feeling the fatigue from a hard run, tap your shirt 3 times and inhale. There are powerful oxygen molecules released that will help to revive your muscles.

- **Bouncy air pads on your feet**
  During the last third of your race, when you feel that the feet aren't bouncing any more, turn on the mental switch that inserts air into the skin on the bottom of your feet. It is only activated if you shorten your stride and keep your feet low to the ground.

Note: In our book *Mental Training for Runners*, you'll find the mental coaching for the following situations:

- Getting out the door early in the morning

- Getting out the door after work, school, a tough day

- Finishing a tough workout

- Doing the next segment

- Finishing a tough race

- Coming back from an injury

- Coming back from an illness

- Coming back from an extended layoff

- Coming back after a bad race or workout

- Burning more fat

- A close running friend moves away, etc.

- Reprogramming the reflex brain to use Run-Walk-Run

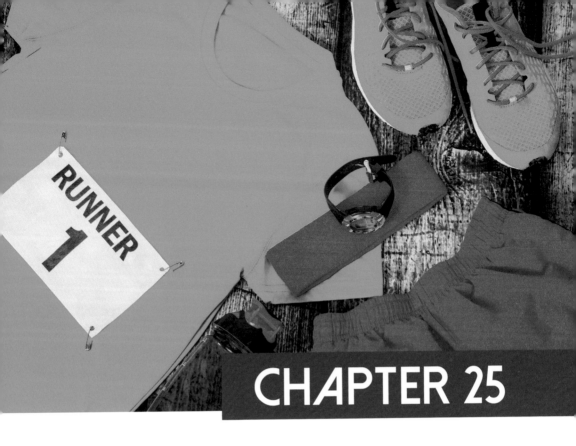

CHAPTER 25

DESTROYING EXCUSES

All of us have days when we don't feel like running. On some of those days you probably need a day off due to too much running or other physical activity. But usually this is not the case. The fact is that when we are under stress in life (and who isn't), the subconscious reflex brain triggers negative attitude hormones when we think of adding workout stress. Each of us can choose whether to listen to the excuse or not. Once you quickly decide whether there is a medical (or other legitimate reason) why you shouldn't run, most of the time you'll shift control to the conscious brain and override the negativity of the reflex.

Thinking ahead will not take any significant time away from your day, and will destroy most of these excuses.

You'll discover pockets of time, more energy, quality time with kids, and more enjoyment from exercise than you thought possible.

The following is a list of excuses that most of us hear on a regular basis. With each, I've given a strategy for breaking through the excuse. Most of the time, it is as simple as just getting out the door and getting your feet moving. But overall, you are the captain of

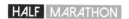
your ship. If you take charge over your schedule and your attitude, you will plan ahead. This gets you into the executive brain and can allow you to focus on positive forward motion. Put one foot in front of the other, the endorphins start flowing, and the excuses start to melt away. Life is good!

"I DON'T HAVE TIME TO RUN"

Most of the recent US presidents have been runners, as well as most of their vice presidents. Are you busier than the president? There are always pockets of time, 5 minutes here, 10 minutes there, when you can insert a walk-run. With planning, you'll find several half-hours each week. Many runners find that as they get in better shape, they don't need as much sleep, which allows for a chunk of time before the day gets started. It all gets down to the question, "Are you going to take control over the organization of your day or not?" Once you look at your schedule, you'll usually discover other time blocks that allow you to do other things. By making time for a run, you will also tend to be more productive and efficient, more than "paying back" the time you spend running. The bottom line is that you have the time – take it and you will have more quality in your life.

"THE RUN WILL HURT OR MAKE ME TIRED"

If this happens, you are the one responsible. You have almost complete control over both of these outcomes. By going at a conservative pace, with the right amount of running and walking, you will feel better and more energized after the run than before.

If you have a bad habit of pushing the pace too much in the beginning, then get control over yourself! Walk more in the beginning, and slow down your running pace. As you learn to slow down, you'll avoid pain and come away from the run with more energy.

"I NEED TO SPEND SOME TIME WITH MY KIDS"

There are a number of running strollers that allow parents to run with their kids. The two of us logged thousands of miles with our first child in single "baby jogger." We got a twin carrier after our second was born. With the right pacing, you can talk to the kids about anything, and they can't run or crawl away.

Sorry, they don't have a model for teenagers. Because you are with the kid(s) in close company, we found that we talked more, and got more feedback than doing other activities together. By bringing them along with you on a run, you become a great role model: even though you're busy, you take time to exercise and spend time with your kids.

"I'VE GOT TOO MUCH WORK TO DO"

There will always be work to do. Several surveys have found that runners get more work done on days they run. Running activates brain circuits that improve attitude and vitality, while reducing stress. Hundreds of runners have told me that the early morning run allowed the time and mental energy to organize their day better than any other activity.

Others said that the after-work run relieved stress and tied up the mental loose ends from the office. Clearly you will get as much (probably more) work done each day if you run regularly. It is up to you to take charge so that you will insert the run into your day.

"I DON'T HAVE THE ENERGY TO RUN TODAY"

This is one of the easier ones to dissolve. Most of the runners who've worked with me and had this excuse had not been managing their blood sugar level (BSL). By writing down what you eat, you can keep your BSL stable. You will also avoid reflex eating, which results in putting more fat on the body. By eating about every 2-3 hours, most people feel more energized, more often. Even if you aren't eating well during the day, you can overcome low blood sugar by having a "booster" snack about an hour before a run. Caffeine helps (as long as you don't have caffeine sensitivities).

My dynamic food duo is an energy bar and a cup of coffee. Just carry some food with you and energize yourself before a run. On trips, I carry packets of instant coffee so that I can have a cup of coffee almost anywhere.

"I DON'T HAVE MY RUNNING SHOES AND CLOTHES WITH ME"

Take an old bag (backpack, etc.) and load it with a pair of running shoes, a top for both winter and summer, shorts and warm-up pants, towel, deodorant, and anything else you would need for a run and clean-up. Put the bag next to the front door, or in the trunk of your car, etc. Then, the next time you are waiting to pick up your child from soccer, etc, you can do a quick change in the restroom and make some loops around the field.

"I'D RATHER BE SITTING ON A COUCH EATING CANDY"

Ok, now it's time for your "test." What is your response to this type of message?

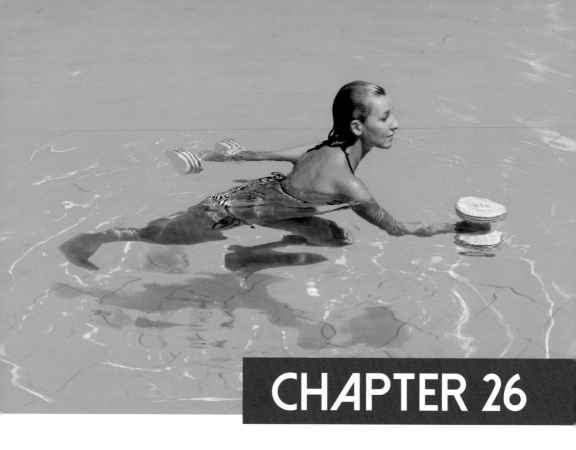

CHAPTER 26

CROSS-TRAINING: EXERCISE FOR THE NON-RUNNING DAYS

My run-walk method has helped tens of thousands of new runners avoid injury while enjoying the increased vitality and attitude improvement that comes with regular running.

A growing percentage of these new runners have had such a good experience with running injury free that they think they are immune to aches and pains. They are wrong.

TOO MUCH OF *A* GOOD THING

When you run, you must lift your body weight off the ground and then absorb the shock as it comes back down. If you are doing this every other day, the limited damage can almost always be repaired and your fitness improved. Many runners, even in their 50s and 60s, don't ever have lingering problems.

Once runners get into a regular running routine and enjoy the vitality and attitude boost, some will try to sneak in an extra day or two on the days they should be resting the running muscles. The same people who had trouble getting motivated for months suddenly get out of control and suffer from aches and pains. The logic goes like this: if the minimal amount of running made them feel pretty good, increasing the mileage has to make them feel much better. The reality is that when adding one or two extra running days, the injury risk doubles or triples.

> **Note:** If you are running more often than every other day and not having problems, it's fine to continue. But at the first sign of lingering fatigue or irritation of a weak link, run every 48 hours.

CROSS-TRAINING ACTIVITIES

The middle ground is to run one day and cross train the next. Cross-training simply means "alternative exercise" to running. Your goal is to find exercises that give you an exercise boost while allowing the running muscles to recover and rebuild: calf, Achilles tendon, ankle, foot.

The other exercises may not deliver the same good feelings, but they can come close. Many runners report that it may take a combination of 3 or 4 different ones in a session. But even if you don't feel exactly the same way, you'll receive the relaxation that comes from exercise, while burning calories and fat.

WHEN YOU ARE STARTING TO DO ANY EXERCISE (OR STARTING AFTER A LAYOFF):

- Start with 5 easy minutes of each exercise, rest for 20 or more minutes and do 5 more easy minutes.
- You may do 3-5 different exercises during a cross-training session if they don't use the same muscles.
- Take a day of rest after this type of exercise (you can do another exercise the next day).
- Increase by 2-3 additional minutes on each exercise, each session until you get to the number of minutes that you feel comfortable doing.
- Once you have reached two 15-minute sessions, you could shift to one 22-25-minute session and increase by 2-3 more minutes per session if you wish.
- It's best to do no exercise the day before a long run.
- To maintain your conditioning in each exercise it's best to do one session a week of 10 minutes or more once you reach that amount.
- The maximum cross-training is up to the individual. As long as you are feeling fine for the rest of the day and having no trouble with your runs, the length of your cross-training should not be a problem.

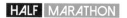

WATER RUNNING CAN IMPROVE RUNNING FORM

All of us have little flips and side motions of our legs that interfere with our running efficiency. The resistance of the water forces your legs to find a more efficient path. In addition, several leg muscles are strengthened, which can help to keep your legs on a smoother path when they get tired at the end of a long run.

HERE'S HOW!

You'll need a flotation belt for this exercise. The product "Aqua Jogger" is designed to float you off the bottom of the pool, and on most runners, tightens so that it is close to the body. There are many other ways to keep you floating, including simple ski float belts and life jackets.

Get in the deep end of the pool and move your legs through a running motion: little or no knee lift, kicking out slightly in front of you, and bringing the leg behind, with the foot coming up so that the lower and upper leg make a 90-degree angle behind you. As in running, your lower leg should be parallel with the horizon.

If you are not feeling much exertion, you're probably lifting the knees too high and moving your legs through a tiny range of motion. To get the benefit, an extended running motion is needed.

It's important to do water running once a week to keep the adaptations that you have gained. If you miss a week, you should drop back a few minutes from your previous session. If you miss more than 3 weeks, start back at two 5-8 min sessions.

FAT BURNING AND OVERALL FITNESS EXERCISES

NORDIC TRACK

This exercise machine simulates the motion used in cross-country skiing. It is one of the better cross-training modes for fat burning because it allows you to use a large number of muscle cells while raising body temperature. If you exercise at an easy pace, you can get into the fat burning zone (past 45 minutes) after a gradual build up to that amount. This exercise requires no pounding of the legs or feet and (unless you push it too hard or too long) allows you to run as usual the next day.

ELLIPTICAL MACHINE

This non-pounding exercise mode is a good cross-training mode. If you need a rest day from running, you should not push hard.

ROWING MACHINE

There are a number of different types of rowing machines. Some work the legs a bit too hard for runners, but most allow you to use a wide variety of lower and upper body muscle groups. Like the Nordic track, if you have the right machine for you, it's possible to continue to exercise for about as long as you wish, once you have gradually worked up to this. Most of the better machines will use a large number of muscle cells, raise the body temperature, and can be continued for more than three-quarters of an hour so they're fat burners.

CYCLING

Indoor cycling (on an exercise cycle) is a better fat burner exercise than outdoor cycling because it raises your body temperature a bit more. The muscles used in both indoor and outdoor cycling are mostly the quadriceps muscles (on the front of the upper thigh), reducing the total number of muscle cells in use compared with the two other modes.

DON'T FORGET WALKING!

Walking can be done all day long, burning a significant number of calories each day. I call walking a "stealth fat-burner" exercise because it is so easy to walk mile after mile, especially in small doses. But it is also an excellent cross-training exercise (this includes walking on the treadmill).

CROSS-TRAINING FOR THE UPPER BODY

WEIGHT TRAINING

While weight work does not directly benefit running, it can be done on non-running days or on running days (after a run). There is a wide range of different ways to build strength. If interested, find a coach who can help you build strength in the muscle groups you wish. Before doing any strength exercise, including the ones in this book, make sure that you don't have any orthopedic issues related to each exercise. As mentioned previously, weight training for the legs is not recommended.

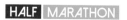

POSTURAL MUSCLE EXERCISE

We recommend two exercises to maintain good postural strength. These will give you a platform of strength to keep you upright and balanced for running, and for life. The wide range of muscles strengthened by these exercises can help support the spine and neck. Many heavy-chested women who have a tendency to lean forward and experience back or neck pain have experienced great benefit from doing these exercises. It is recommended that you do these exercises 2-3 days per week.

The Crunch – Lying on your back, with knees bent, move your head and shoulders slightly off the floor and ease back down. Keep moving in this narrow range of motion for 5-10 seconds at first, take a rest of a minute or two and repeat 3 to 5 times. Gradually increase the duration of each crunch to 15-20 seconds each.

Arm Running – With hand-held weights (dumbells) in the standing position (not while running), move your arms in slow motion through a range of motion that is similar to what you would use when running. Keep the weights close to the body as you move them from waist to shoulders and down. Start with 3 sets of four or five and gradually increase to 3-5 sets of 10. Choose a weight that gives you a feeling that you have strengthened the muscles without having to struggle to do the ninth and tenth repetitions.

SWIMMING

While not a fat-burner, swimming strengthens the upper body while improving cardiovascular fitness and endurance in those muscles. Swimming can be done on both running and non-running days.

DON'T DO THESE ON NON-RUNNING DAYS!

The following exercises will tire the muscles used for running and keep them from recovering between run days. If you really like to do any of these exercises, you can do them after a run on a running day.

- Stair machines
- Stair aerobics
- Weight training for the leg muscles
- Power walking – especially on a hilly course
- Spinning classes (on a bicycle) in which you get out of your seat

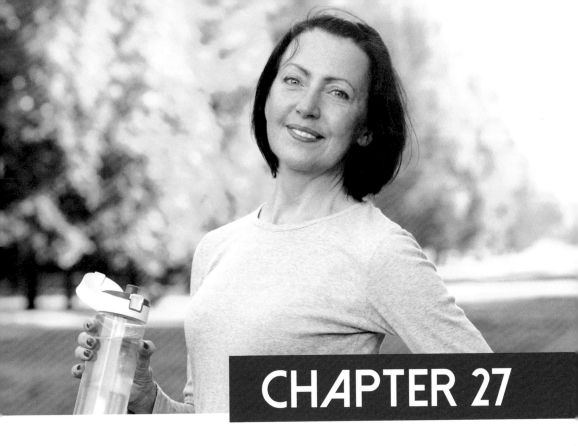

CHAPTER 27

DEALING WITH THE WEATHER

"Neither rain, nor ice, nor heat, nor gloom, nor night shall keep us from our run."

Sometimes, on the snowy, rainy, brutally cold or hot days, I yearn for the early days of running when we had an excuse for not braving the elements. Today, however, there are garments for each of the above, head to toe. Yes, technology has taken away most of our excuses for not exercising. But runners can be very creative. Every year I hear a few new ones from those who rise to the occasion and find some reason why they can't exercise. But even if you don't have the clothing for hot or cold weather, you can run/walk indoors on treadmills, in malls or stadiums, or at a gym.

A few years ago, I ran a race in Fairbanks, Alaska. I had to ask the members of the local running club what was the lowest temperature anyone had endured. The winner had run a 10K in minus 66 (not wind chill, this was the real thing: bulb temperature). He said that it really didn't feel that cold.

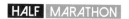

The fact is that clothing designers have responded to the needs of runners during extreme weather conditions, making it possible to run, fairly comfortably, in sub-zero conditions. I will admit, however, that if it is minus 66, I can't run because I have to rearrange my running shoes next to a warm fire.

HOT WEATHER

I've heard rumors of an air-conditioned suit for the heat, but haven't seen it offered by the clothing manufacturers. I could have used this when I ran a marathon in Key West, Florida, when it was 95 degrees for the last 20 miles of the race. After decades of running in hot weather areas, mostly in Florida and Georgia, with some time spent in Hawaii and the Philippines, I haven't seen much in clothing that lowers body temperature.

The best you can hope for is to minimize the rise, while you feel cooler, and a bit more comfortable.

When you exercise strenuously in high heat (above 70F/19C), or moderate heat (above 60F/14C) with high humidity (for the individual), core body temperature will rise. Most beginning runners will see the internal temperature rise when the outside temperature goes above 55F (12C). This triggers a release of blood into the capillaries of your skin to help cool you down. But this diversion reduces the blood supply available to your exercising muscles meaning that you will have less blood and less oxygen delivered to the power source that moves you forward and less blood to move out the waste products from these work sites.

So the bad news is that in warm weather you are going to feel worse and run slower. If you build up the heat too quickly, stay out too long, or run too fast – for you – the result could be heat disease. Make sure that you read the section on this health problem at the end of this chapter. The good news is that you can adapt to these conditions to some extent as you learn the best time of the day, clothing to wear, and other tricks to keep you cool. But there are some other good options following, so read on.

RUNNING THROUGH THE SUMMER HEAT

- Run before the sun gets above the horizon. Get up early during warm weather and you will significantly reduce the dramatic stress increase due to sunlight. This is particularly a problem in humid areas. Early morning is usually the coolest time of the day, also. Without having to deal with the sun, most runners can gradually adapt to heat. At the very least, your runs will be more enjoyable. Note: be sure to take care of safety issues.

- If you must run when the sun is up, pick a shady course. Shade provides significant relief in areas of low humidity and some relief in humid environments.

- Evening and night running is usually cooler in areas with low humidity. In humid environments, there may not be much relief.

- Have an indoor facility available. With treadmills, you can exercise in air conditioning. If a treadmill bores you, alternate segments of 5-10 minutes – one segment outdoors and the next indoors.

- Don't wear a hat! You lose most of your body heat through the top of your head. Covering the head will cause a quicker internal build-up of heat.

- Wear light clothing but not cotton. Many of the new, technical fibers (Polypro, Coolmax, Drifit, DryScience, etc.) will move moisture away from your skin, producing a cooling effect. Cotton soaks up the sweat, making the garment heavier without providing much of a cooling effect.

- Pour water over your head. Evaporation not only helps the cooling process, it makes you feel cooler. If you can bring along ice water with you, you will feel a lot cooler as you squirt some regularly over the top of your head. I like to freeze an ifitness belt bottle half full, and then fill it up with water as I start my run.

- Do your maintenance runs in installments. It is fine, on a hot day, to put in your 30 minutes by doing 10 in the morning, 10 at noon, and 10 at night. The long run, however, should be done at one time.

- Take a pool break or a shower chill-down. During a run, it really helps to take a 2-4 minute dip in a pool or a shower. Some runners in hot areas run loops around their neighborhood and let the hose run over their head each lap. The pool is especially helpful in soaking out excess body temperature. I have run in 97-degree temperatures at our Florida retreat area, breaking up a 5-mile run into 3 x 1.7 mi. Between each, I take a 2-3 minute "soak break" and get back out there. It was only at the end of each segment that I felt hot again.

- Sunscreen – be sure to protect yourself. Some products, however, produce a coating on the skin, slowing down the production and evaporation of perspiration and causing an increase in body temperature build-up. If you are only in the sun for 10-30 minutes at a time, you may not need to put on sunscreen for cancer protection. Consult with a dermatologist for your specific needs or find a product that doesn't block the pores.

- Drink 6-8 oz of a sports drink like Accelerade or water at least every 2 hours, or when thirsty, throughout the day during hot weather.

- Look at the clothing thermometer at the end of this book. Wear loose fitting garments that have some texture in the fabric. Texture will limit or prevent the perspiration from clinging and sticking to the skin.

- If your only option is going outside on a very hot day, you have my permission to rearrange your running shoes – preferably in front of the air conditioning vent.

HOT WEATHER SLOWDOWN

As the temperature rises above 55F(12C), your body starts to build up heat, but most runners aren't significantly slowed until 60F (14C). If you make the adjustments early, you may not suffer later and slow down dramatically at that time. The baseline for this table is 60F or 14C.

Between 60F and 65F – slow down 30 seconds/mile slower than you would run at 60F

Between 14C and 17C – slow down 20 seconds/kilometer than you would run at 14C

Between 66F and 69F – slow down one minute/mile slower than you would run at 60F

Between 18C and 19C – slow down 40 seconds/kilometer slower than you would run at 14C

Between 70F and 75F – slow down 1:30/mile slower than you would run at 60F

Between 19C and 22C – slow down one minute/kilometer slower than you would run at 14C

Between 76F and 80F – slow down 2 min/mile slower than you would run at 60F

Between 23C and 25C – slow down 1:20/kilometer slower than you would run at 14C

Above 80F and 25C –   be careful, take extra precautions to avoid heat disease

Or ... exercise indoors

Or ... arrange your shoes next to the air conditioner

HEAT DISEASE ALERT!

While it is unlikely that you will push yourself into heat disease, the longer you exercise in hot (or humid) conditions, the more you increase the likelihood of this dangerous medical situation. That's why I recommend breaking up your exercise into short segments when it's hot and you must run outdoors. Be sensitive to your reactions to the heat, and those of the runners around you. When one of the symptoms is present, this is normally not a major problem unless there is significant distress. But when several are experienced, take action because heat disease can lead to death. It's always better to be conservative: stop the workout and cool off.

SYMPTOMS:

- Intense heat build-up in the head
- General overheating of the body
- Significant headache
- Significant nausea or vomiting
- General confusion and loss of concentration
- Loss of muscle control
- Excessive sweating and then cessation of sweating
- Clammy skin
- Excessively rapid breathing
- Muscle cramps
- Feeling faint
- Diarrhea
- Vomiting

RISK FACTORS:

- Viral or bacterial infection
- Taking medication – especially cold medicines, diuretics, medicines for diarrhea, antihistamines, atropine, scopolamine, tranquilizers
- Dehydration (especially due to alcohol)
- Severe sunburn
- Overweight
- Lack of heat training
- Exercising more than one is used to
- Occurrence of heat disease in the past
- Several nights of extreme sleep deprivation
- Certain medical conditions, including high cholesterol, high blood pressure, extreme stress, asthma, diabetes, epilepsy, drug use (including alcohol), cardiovascular disease, smoking, or a general lack of fitness

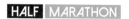

TAKE ACTION! CALL 911

Use your best judgement, but in most cases, anyone who exhibits two or more of those symptoms should get into a cool environment and receive medical attention immediately. An extremely effective cool-off method is to soak towels, sheets, or clothing in cool or cold water and wrap them around the individual. If ice is available, sprinkle some ice over the wet cloth.

> ### TIP: MAINTAINING HEAT TOLERANCE DURING THE WINTER
>
> By putting on additional layers of clothing so that you sweat within 3-4 minutes of your run-walk, you can keep much of your summer heat conditioning that took so much work to produce. Continue to run for a total of 5-12 minutes at an easy pace. Don't let yourself get too hot so that you experience heat disease symptoms.

DEALING WITH THE COLD

While most of my runs have been in temperatures above 60F, I've also run in minus-30. I prepared for this run extensively and put on about as many layers as I had in my suitcase. My winter running guide quickly evaluated my clothing and found me lacking. After another two layers, I was ready to go.

The specific type of garments, especially the one next to your skin, is an individual issue. Be sure to look at the "Clothing Thermometer" at the end of this book as a guide for dressing according to the temperature. In general, you want your first layer to be comfortable and not too thick. There are a number of technical fabrics today, mostly man-made, that hold a comfortable amount of body heat close to the skin to keep you warm but don't let you overheat. Most of these same fibers allow for moisture, such as perspiration and rain, to be moved away from the skin – even as you run and walk. Not only does this add to your comfort in winter but chill from wet skin is significantly reduced or eliminated.

RUNNING THROUGH THE CHILL OF WINTER

- Expand your lunch hour if you want to run outdoors. Midday is usually the warmest time of the day, so you will probably have to plan to arrive at work early (paper work, run errands, etc.). The midday sun can make your outdoor running much more comfortable, even when it is very cold.

- If early morning is the only time you can run, bundle up. The "Clothing Thermometer" at the end of this book will help you to dress for the temperature and not over dress.

- Run into the wind at the start, particularly when you are running out and turning around. If you run with the wind at your back for the first half of the run, you'll tend to sweat. When you turn into a cold wind, you'll chill dramatically.

- Having a health club will give you an indoor venue and other exercise options. With treadmills, you can run away from the wind chill. I have worked with many runners who hate running on treadmills but also hate running for more than 15 minutes in the cold. Their solution is to alternate segments of 7-15 minutes – one segment outdoors and the next indoors. Count the transition as a walk break. Health clubs expand your exercise horizons by offering a variety of alternative exercise.

- One of your exercise days could be a triathlon – your choice of three exercises. You can do exercises out of your home or at a health club. See the sidebar on "Winter triathlon" for more information.

- Seek out a large indoor facility near your office or home. In Houston, runners use the tunnels below city streets. Many northern cities offer skyways and allow runners and walkers to use them when traffic allows it. Domes, malls, and civic centers often allow winter runners and walkers at certain times.

- Wear a hat! You lose most of your body heat through the top of your head. Covering the head will help you retain body heat and stay warm.

- Cover your extremities from the wind chill you produce when you run and walk in the cold! Protect ears, hands, nose, and generally the front of the face. Make sure that you protect the feet with socks that are thick enough.

- Do your run-walk in installments. It is fine, on a really cold day, to put in your 30 minutes by doing 10 in the morning, 10 at noon, and 10 at night.

- Take a "warm-up" break. Before you head out into the cold, walk and run in place indoors. During a run, when you get really cold on the outside, it really helps to take a 2-4 minute walk indoors. Some runners schedule their walk breaks to coincide with buildings that allow public walking.

- Vaseline – be sure to protect yourself wherever there is exposed skin on very cold days. One area, for example, is the skin around the eyes that is not protected by a ski mask, etc.

- When you are exercising during the winter, indoors or outdoors, you will be losing almost as much in sweat as in the warm months. You should still drink at least 4-6 oz of a sports drink like Accelerade, two or three times a day. In addition, I recommend consuming 5-6 glasses of water or juice each day. During a long run, the recommended fluid intake is 2-4 oz (60-120ml) of water every 20-25 minutes.

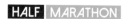

WINTER TRIATHLON

Energize your winter workouts by doing three or more segments during your training. Here's how it works:

- Select one day a week for your triathlon. Choose three activities.

- Outdoor activities: run-walk, cross-country skiing, skating, snowshoeing, etc.

- Indoor health club activities: run-walk, swim, stair machine, exercycle, rowing machine, etc.

- Indoor activities at home: exercise machines, stairs, weights, sit-ups, rope skipping, running in place, aerobic video exercise.

- Alternate the activities for about 5-10 minutes at a time.

- If desired, keep a log of how much work you do on each machine, miles run, minutes for each activity, etc.

- Expand to a pentathlon (5 events), decathlon (10 events) or whatever.

- Combine indoor and outdoor activities if you wish – set up your "world record" list.

- Challenge your friends – even if they live in different cities – compare notes by email.

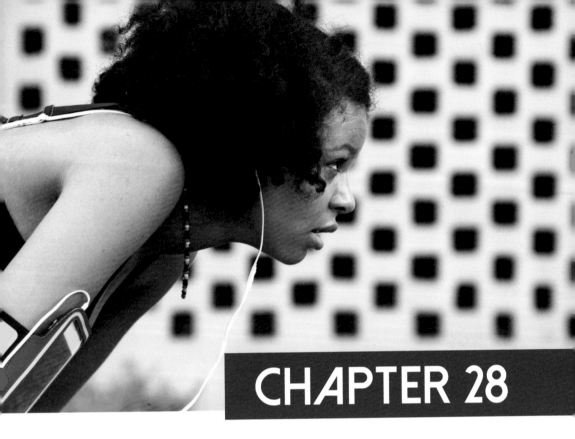

CHAPTER 28

TROUBLESHOOTING

- Coming back after a layoff from running
- It hurts!
- No energy
- Side pain
- I feel great one day – but the next day...
- No motivation
- Cramps in my leg muscles
- Upset stomach or diarrhea
- Headache
- Should I run when I have a cold?
- Street safety
- Dogs
- Heart disease and running

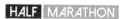

HOW DO I START BACK WHEN I'VE HAD TIME OFF?

The longer you've been away from running, the slower you must return. I want to warn you now that you will reach a point when you feel totally back in shape, but you are not. Stay with the following plan for your return and when in doubt, be more conservative. Remember that you are in this for the long run!

Less than 2 weeks off – You will feel like you are starting over again but should come back quickly. Let's say that you were at week 10, but had to take 10 days off. Start back at week 2 for the first week. If all is well, skip to week 3 or 4 for the second week. If that works well, gradually transition back to the schedule you were using before you had your layoff over the next 2-3 weeks.

14 days to 29 days off – You will also feel like you are starting over again, and it will take longer to get it all back. Within about 5-6 weeks you should be back to normal. Use the schedule of your choice (from week 1) for two weeks. If there are no aches, pains, or lingering fatigue, then use the schedule but skip every other week. After the fifth week, transition back into what you were doing before the layoff.

One month or more off – If you have not run for a month or more, start over again like a beginner. Use one of the three schedules in this book, following it exactly (from week 1) for the first few weeks. After 2-3 weeks, the safest plan is to continue with the schedule. But if you're having no aches or pains and no lingering fatigue, you could increase more rapidly by skipping one week out of three. After 2 months of no problems, your conditioning can often be back to pre-injury levels.

IT HURTS! IS IT JUST *A* PASSING *A*CHE OR *A* REAL INJURY?

Most of the aches and pains you feel when running will go away within a minute or two. If the pain comes on when running, just walk for an additional 2 minutes, jog a few strides, and walk another 2 minutes. If the pain comes back after doing this 4 or 5 times, stop running and walk. If the pain goes away when you walk, just walk for the rest of the workout.

Walking pain – When the pain stays around when walking, try a very short stride. Walk for a 30-60 seconds. If it still hurts when walking, try sitting down and massaging the area that hurts (if you can). Sit for 2-4 minutes. If you try again to walk and it still hurts, call it a day – your workout is over.

It's an injury if ...

There's inflammation – swelling in the area

There's loss of function – the foot, knee, etc., doesn't work correctly

There's pain – it hurts and keeps hurting or gets worse

TREATMENT SUGGESTIONS:

- See a doctor who has treated other runners very successfully and wants to get you back on the road or trail.

- Take at least 2-5 days off from any activity that could irritate it to get the healing started, more if needed.

- If the injury site is next to the skin (tendon, foot, etc.), rub a chunk of ice on the area(s), constantly rubbing for 15 min until the area gets numb. Continue to do this for a week after you feel no symptoms. Ice bags and gel ice do no good at all in most cases.

- If the problem is inside a joint or muscle, call your doctor and ask if you can use prescription strength anti-inflammatory medication. Don't take any medication without a doctor's advice, and follow that advice.

- If you have a muscle injury, see a veteran sports massage therapist. Try to find one who has a lot of successful experience treating the area where you are injured. The magic fingers and hands can often work wonders.

This is advice from one runner to another. For more info on injuries, treatment, etc., see a doctor and read *Injuries – Care and Prevention* by Dr. David Hannaford and myself.

> **Note:** The best treatment I've found for exhausted or irritated soft tissue is the BFF vibrating massage tool, which you can buy from www.JeffGalloway.com. The vibration action invigorates muscles and tendons and increases blood flow. Those who attend my running schools, retreats, and training programs receive a discount.

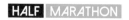

NO ENERGY TODAY

There will be a number of days each year when you will not feel like exercising. On most of these, you can turn it around and feel great. Occasionally, you will not be able to do this because of an infection, lingering fatigue, or other physical problems. Here's a list of things that can give you energy. If these actions don't lead you to a run, then read the nutrition sections – particularly the blood sugar chapter in this book, or *Running and Fat Burning for Women*.

- Eat an energy bar with water or caffeinated beverage, about 30 minutes before the run. Caffeine helps!

- Or, half an hour before exercising, you could drink 100-200 calories of a sports drink that has a mix of 80% simple carbohydrate and 20% protein. The product Accelerade already has this ratio.

- Just walk for 5 minutes away from your house, office, etc., and the energy often kicks in. Forward movement gets the attitude moving, too.

- One of the prime reasons for no energy is that you didn't reload within 30 minutes after your last exercise session: 200-300 calories of a mix that is 80% simple carbohydrate and 20% protein (Endurox R4 is the product that has this formulation).

- Low-carb diets will result in low energy to get motivated before a workout and often no energy to finish the workout.

- In most cases, it is fine to keep going even if you aren't energetic. But if you sense an infection, see a doctor. If the low energy stays around for several days, see a nutritionist who knows about the special needs of exercisers or get some bloodwork done. The lack of energy may be due to inadequate iron, B vitamins, energy stores, etc.

Note: If you have any problems with caffeine, don't consume any products containing it. As always, if you sense any health problem, see a doctor.

SIDE PAIN

This is very common and usually has a simple fix. Normally, it is not anything to worry about, it just hurts. This condition is due to 1) the lack of lower lung breathing, and 2) going a little too fast from the beginning of the run. You can correct number 2 easily by walking more at the beginning and slowing down your running pace.

Lower lung breathing from the beginning of a run has prevented side pain in a high percentage of cases I've seen. This way of inhaling air is performed by diverting the air you breathe into your lower lungs. Also called "belly breathing," this is how we breathe when asleep, and it provides the maximum opportunity for oxygen absorption. If you don't do this from the beginning of a run, you are not getting the oxygen you need – the side pain will tell you. By slowing down, walking, and breathing deeply for a while, the pain may go away.

But sometimes it does not. Most runners just continue to run and walk with the side pain. In over 50 years of running and helping others run, I've not seen any lasting negative effect from those who run with a side pain.

You don't have to take in a maximum breath to perform this technique. Simply breathe a normal breath but send it to the lower lungs. You know that you have done this if your stomach goes up and down as you inhale and exhale. If your chest goes up and down, you are breathing shallowly.

Note: Never breathe in and out rapidly. This can lead to hyperventilation, dizziness, and fainting.

I FEEL GREAT ONE DAY ... AND NOT THE NEXT

If you can solve this problem, you could become a very wealthy person. There are a few common reasons for this, but there will always be "those days" when the body doesn't seem to work right – the gravity seems heavier than normal – and you cannot find a reason.

- Pushing through. In most cases, this is a one-day occurrence. Most runners just put more walking into the mix and get through it. Before pushing, however, make sure that you don't have a medical reason why you feel bad. Don't exercise when you have a lung infection, for example.

- Heat and humidity will make you feel worse. You will often feel great when the temperature is below 60F and miserable when 80F or above (especially at the end of the workout).

- Low blood sugar can make any run a bad run. You may feel good at the start and suddenly feel like you have no energy. Every step seems to take a major effort. Read the chapter in this book about this topic.

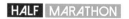

- Low motivation. Use the rehearsal techniques in the "staying motivated" chapter to get you out the door on a bad day. These have helped numerous runners turn their minds around, even in the middle of a run.

- Infection can leave you feeling lethargic, achy, and unable to run at the same pace that was easy a few days earlier. Check the normal signs (fever, chills, swollen lymph glands, etc.) and at least call your doctor if you suspect something.

- Medication and alcohol, even when taken the day before, can leave a hangover that dampens a workout.

- A slower start can make the difference between a good day and a bad day. When your body is on the edge of fatigue or other stress, it only takes a few seconds too fast per mile, walking or running, to push into discomfort or worse.

CRAMPS IN THE MUSCLES

At some point, most people who run experience cramps. These muscle contractions usually occur in the feet or the calf muscles and may come during a run or walk, or they may hit at random. Most commonly, they will occur at night or when you are sitting around at your desk or watching TV in the afternoon or evening.

Cramps vary in severity. Most are mild but some can grab so hard that they shut down the muscles and hurt when they seize up. Massage, and a short and gentle movement of the muscle, can help to bring most of the cramps around. Odds are that stretching will make the cramp worse or tear the muscle fibers.

Most cramps are due to overuse – exercising farther or faster than in the recent past or continuing to put yourself at your limit, especially in warm weather. Look at the pace and distance of your runs and walks in your training journal to see if you have been running too far, too fast, or both.

- Continuous running increases cramping. Taking walk breaks more often can reduce or eliminate cramps. Many runners who used to cramp when they ran a minute and walked a minute stopped cramping with a ratio of run 30 seconds and walk 30-60 seconds.

- During hot weather, a good electrolyte beverage can help replace the salts that you body loses in sweating. A drink like Accelerade, for example, can help to top off these minerals when you drink approximately 6-8 oz every 1-2 hours.

- On very long hikes, walks or runs, however, the continuous sweating, especially when drinking a lot of fluid, can push your sodium levels too low and produce muscle cramping. If you are mostly walking and are still experiencing cramps, the buffered salt tablet, succeed, can help grently.

- Many medications, especially those designed to lower cholesterol, list muscle cramps as one of their known side effects. Runners who use medications and cramp up should ask their doctor if there are alternatives.

HERE ARE SEVERAL WAYS OF DEALING WITH CRAMPS:

- Take a longer and more gentle warm-up

- Shorten your run segment

- Slow down your walk and walk more

- Shorten your distance on a hot/humid day

- Break your run up into two segments

- Look at any other exercise that could be causing the cramps

- Take a buffered salt tablet at the beginning of your exercise

- Shorten your stride – especially on hills

Note: If you have high blood pressure, ask your doctor before taking any salt product.

UPSET STOMACH OR DIARRHEA

Sooner or later, virtually every runner has at least one episode with nausea or diarrhea (N/D). It comes from the build-up of total stress that you accumulate. Most commonly, it is the stress of running on that day due to the causes listed next. But stress can come from many unique conditions within the individual. Your body triggers the N/D to get you to reduce the exercise, which will reduce the stress. Here are the common causes:

- **Running too fast or too far is the most common cause.** Runners are confused about this because the pace doesn't feel too fast in the beginning. Each person has a level of fatigue that triggers these conditions. Slowing down and taking more walk breaks will help you manage the problem.

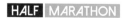

- **Eating too much or too soon before the run.** Your system has to work hard when you're running and works hard to digest food. Doing both at the same time raises stress and results in nausea, etc. Having food in your stomach in the process of being digested is an extra stress and a likely target for elimination.

- **Eating a high-fat or high-protein diet.** Even one meal that has over 50% of the calories in fat or protein can lead to N/D hours later.

- **Eating too much the afternoon or evening on the day before.** A big evening meal will still be in the gut the next morning, being digested. When you bounce up and down on a run, which you will, you add stress to the system often producing N/D.

- **Heat and humidity** are a major cause of these problems. Some people don't adapt to heat well and experience N/D with minimal build-up of temperature or humidity. But in hot conditions, everyone has a core body temperature increase that will result in significant stress to the system – often causing nausea and sometimes diarrhea. By slowing down, taking more walk breaks, and pouring water over your head, you can manage this better. The best time to exercise in warm weather is before the sun gets above the horizon.

- **Drinking too much water *before* a run.** If you have too much water in your stomach and you are bouncing around, you put stress on the digestive system. Reduce your intake to the bare minimum. Most runners don't need to drink any fluid before a run that is 60 minutes or less.

- **Drinking too much of a sugar/electrolyte drink.** Water is the easiest substance for the body to process. The addition of sugar or electrolyte minerals, as in a sports drink, makes the substance harder to digest for many runners. During a run (especially on a hot day), it is best to drink only water. Cold water is best.

- **Drinking too much fluid too soon *after* a run.** Even if you are very thirsty, don't gulp down large quantities of any fluid. Try to drink no more than 6-8 oz every 20 minutes or so. If you are particularly prone to N/D, just take 2-4 sips every 5 minutes or so. When the body is very stressed and tired, it's not a good idea to consume a sugar drink. The extra stress of digesting the sugar can lead to problems.

- **Don't let running be stressful to you.** Some runners get too obsessed about getting their run in or running at a specific pace. This adds stress to your life. Relax and let your run diffuse some of the other tensions in your life.

HEADACHE

There are several reasons why runners get headaches on runs. While uncommon, they happen to the average runner about 1-5 times a year. The extra stress that running puts on the body can trigger a headache on a tough day, even considering the relaxation that comes from the run. Many runners find that a dose of an over-the-counter headache medication takes care of the problem. As always, consult with your doctor about using medication. Here are the causes/solutions:

Dehydration – If you run in the morning, make sure that you hydrate well the day before. Avoid alcohol if you run in the mornings and have headaches. Also watch the salt in your dinner meal the night before. A good sports drink, like Accelerade, taken throughout the day before will help keep your fluid levels and electrolytes "topped off." If you run in the afternoon, follow the same advice leading up to your run on the day of the run.

Medications can often produce dehydration – There are some medications that make runners more prone to headaches. Check with your doctor.

Too hot for you – Run at a cooler time of the day (usually in the morning before the sun gets above the horizon). When on a hot run, pour water over your head.

Pollen, asthma, allergies – At certain times of the year, those who have allergies tend to get headaches. Check with your doctor about inhalers, medication, etc.

Running a little too fast – Start all runs more slowly, walk more during the first half of the run.

Running farther than you have run in the recent past – Monitor your mileage and don't increase more than about 15% farther than you have run on any single run in the past week.

Low blood sugar level – Be sure that you boost your BLS with a snack, about 30-60 min before you run. If you are used to having it, caffeine in a beverage can sometimes help this situation also.

If prone to migraines – Generally avoid caffeine, and try your best to avoid dehydration. Talk to your doctor about other possibilities.

Watch your neck and lower back – If you have a slight forward lean as you run, you can put pressure on the spine (particularly in the neck and lower back). Read the form chapter in this book and run upright.

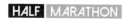

SHOULD I RUN *WHEN I HAVE A* COLD?

There are so many individual health issues with a cold that you must talk with a doctor before you exercise when you have an infection. Usually you will be given the OK to gently exercise. Check with the doctor.

Lung infection – Don't run! A virus in the lungs can move into the heart and kill you. Lung infections are usually indicated by coughing.

Common cold – There are many infections that initially seem to be a normal cold but are not. At least call your doctor's office to get clearance before running. Be sure to explain how much you are running, and what, if any, medication you are taking.

Throat infection and above – Most runners will be given the OK, but check with the doc.

STREET SAFETY

Each year several runners are hit by cars when running. Most of these situations are preventable. Here are the primary reasons they happen and what you can do about them.

- The driver is intoxicated or preoccupied by cell phone, etc.Always be on guard – even when running on the sidewalk or pedestrian trail. Many of the fatal crashes occurred when the driver lost control of the car and came up behind the runner on the wrong side of the road. I know it is wonderful to be on "cruise control" in your right brain, but you can avoid a life-threatening situation if you just keep looking around and anticipate potential dangers.

- The runner dashes across an intersection against the traffic light.
  When running or walking with another person, don't try to follow blindly across an intersection. Runners who quickly sprint across the street without looking are often surprised by cars coming from unexpected directions. The best rule is the one that you heard as a child: When you get to an intersection, stop and see what the traffic situation is. Look both ways, and look both ways again (and again) before crossing. Have an option to bail out of the crossing if a car surprises you from any direction.

- Sometimes, runners wander out into the street as they talk and run.
  One of the very positive aspects of running becomes a negative one, in this case. Yes, chat and enjoy time with your friends. But every runner in a group needs to be responsible for his or her own safety, footing, etc. The biggest mistake I see is that the runners at the back of a group assume that they don't have to be concerned about traffic at all. This lack of concern is a very risky situation.

- In general, be ready to save yourself from a variety of traffic problems by following the rules and any others that apply to specific situations. Even though the rules seem obvious, many runners get hit by cars each year by ignoring them.

- Be constantly aware of vehicular traffic at all times.

- Assume that all drivers are drunk, crazy, or both. When you see a strange movement by a car, be ready to get out of the way.

- Mentally practice running for safety. Get into the practice of thinking ahead at all times, with a plan for that current stretch of road.

- Run as far off the road as you can. If possible, run on a sidewalk or pedestrian trail.

- Run facing traffic. A high percentage of traffic deaths come from those who run with the flow of traffic and do not see the threat from behind.

- Wear reflective gear at night. I've heard the accounts and this apparel has saved lives.

- Take control over your safety – you are the only one on the road who will usually save yourself.

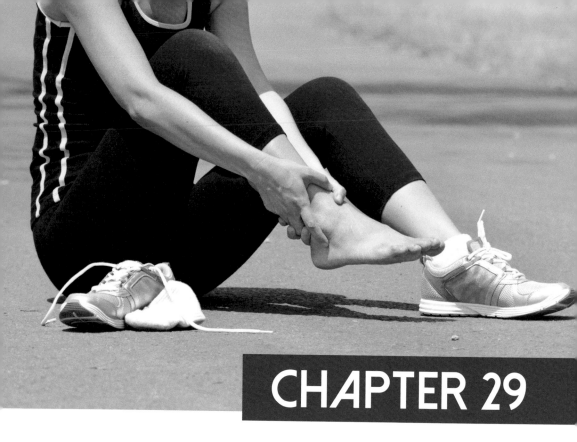

CHAPTER 29

TROUBLESHOOTING ACHES AND PAINS

At the first sign of soreness or irritation in the following areas, read the injury chapter. It is always better to take 2-3 days off from running and then start back making some form adjustments. In most of these "pain sites," I've found that stretching aggravates the problem. For more information, see *Running Injuries – Care and Treatment* and *Galloway's Book on Running, 2nd ed*. Both are available autographed at *www.JeffGalloway.com*.

SHINS, SHOULDER, AND NECK MUSCLES TIRED AND TIGHT

Note: Even after you make corrections, shin problems often take several weeks to heal. As long as the shin problem is not a stress fracture, easy running can often allow it to heal as quickly (or more quickly) than a complete layoff. In general, most runners can run when they have shin splints, they just need to stay below the threshold of further irritation.

SORENESS OR PAIN IN THE FRONT OF THE SHIN (ANTERIOR TIBIAL AREA)

Causes:

- Increasing too rapidly – just walk for 1-2 weeks and walk gently with a short stride.

- Running too fast, even on one day – when in doubt, run slower and walk slower on all runs.

- Running or walking with a stride that is too long – shorten stride and use more of a "shuffle."

SORENESS OR PAIN AT THE INSIDE OF THE LOWER LEG (POSTERIOR TIBIAL AREA)

Causes

- Same three causes as in anterior tibial shin splints.

- More common with runners who over-pronate. This means that they tend to roll to the inside of the foot as they push off.

- Shoes may be too soft, allowing a floppy/pronated foot to roll inward more than usual.

Corrections:

- Reduce stride length.

- Slow the pace at the beginning and insert more walking into your run-walk ratio from the beginning.

- If you are an over-pronator on the forward part of your feet, get a stable, motion control shoe.

- Ask your foot doctor if there is a foot device that can help you.

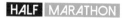

SHOULDER AND NECK

Primary cause: Leaning too far forward as you run.

Other Causes:

- Holding arms too far away from the body as you run.

- Swinging arms and shoulders too much as you run.

Corrections:

- Use the "puppet on a string" image (detailed in the running form chapter) about every 4-5 minutes during all runs and walks – particularly the longer ones. This is noted in the section on posture.

- Watch how you are holding your arms. Try to keep the arms close to the body.

- Minimize the swing of your arms. Keep the hands close to the body, lightly touching your shirt or the outside of your shorts as your arms swing.

LOWER BACK: TIGHT, SORE, OR PAINFUL AFTER A RUN

Causes:

- Leaning too far forward as you run.

- Having a stride length that is too long for you.

Corrections:

- Use the "puppet on a string" image several times on all runs and walks – particularly the longer ones. This is noted in the chapter on running form, in the section on posture.

- Ask a physical therapist whether some strengthening exercises can help.

- When in doubt, shorten your stride length.

- For more information, see *Galloway's Book on Running, second edition*.

KNEE PAIN AT THE END OF A RUN

Causes:

- Stride length could be too long.

- Doing too much, too soon.

- Not inserting enough walk breaks, regularly, from the beginning.

- When the main running muscles get tired, you will tend to wobble from side to side.

Corrections:

- Shorten stride.

- Stay closer to the ground, using more of a shuffle.

- Monitor your mileage in a log book, and hold your increase to less than 10% a week.

- Use more walk breaks during your run.

- Start at a slower pace.

BEHIND THE KNEE: PAIN, TIGHTNESS, OR CONTINUED SORENESS OR WEAKNESS

Causes:

- Stretching.

- Over-striding – particularly at the end of the run.

Corrections:

- Don't stretch.

- Keep your stride length under control.

- Keep feet low to the ground.

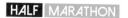

HAMSTRINGS: TIGHTNESS, SORENESS, OR PAIN

Causes:

- Stretching.

- Stride length too long.

- Lifting the foot too high behind, as your leg swings back.

Corrections:

- Don't stretch.

- Maintain a short stride, keeping the hamstring relaxed – especially at the end of the run.

- Take more walk breaks early in the run, possibly throughout the run.

- As the leg swings behind you, let the lower leg rise no higher than a position that is parallel to the horizon before swinging forward again.

- Deep tissue massage can sometimes help with this muscle group.

QUADRICEPS (FRONT OF THE THIGH): SORE, TIRED, PAINFUL

Causes:

- Lifting your knee too high – especially when tired.

- Using the quads to slow down going downhill because you were running too fast.

Corrections:

- Maintain little or no knee lift – especially at the end of your run.

- Run with a shuffle.

- Let your stride get very short at the top of hills, and when tired – don't lengthen it.

- If you are running too fast going down hills, keep shortening stride until you slow down, or take more walk breaks on the downhill.

SORE FEET OR LOWER LEGS

Causes:

- Too much bounce.

- Pushing off too hard.

- Shoes don't fit correctly or are too worn out.

- Insole of shoe is worn out.

Corrections:

- Keep feet low to the ground.

- Maintain a light touch of the feet.

- Get a shoe check to see if your shoes are too worn.

- You may only need a new insole.

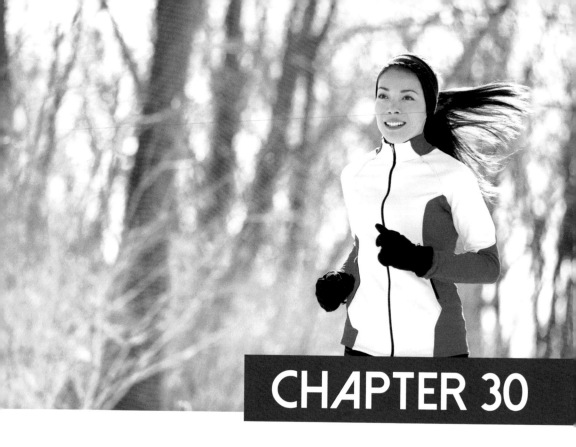

CHAPTER 30

CLOTHING THERMOMETER

After years of working with people in various climates, here are my recommendations for the appropriate clothing based on the temperature. As always, however, wear what works best for you. The general rule is to choose your garments by function first. And remember that the most important layer for comfort is the one next to your skin. Garments made out of fabric labeled Polypro, Coolmax, Drifit, etc. hold enough body heat close to you in winter while releasing extra heat. In summer and winter, they move moisture away from the skin, cooling you in hot weather and avoiding a chill in cold weather.

Temperature	What to wear
60°F and above (14°C+)	Tank top or singlet and shorts
9°C to 13°C or 50 to 59°F	T-shirt and shorts
5 to 8°C or 40 to 49°F	Long-sleeve, lightweight shirt, shorts or tights (or nylon long pants), mittens and gloves
0 to 4°C or 30 to 39°F	Long-sleeve, medium-weight shirt, another T-shirt, tights and shorts, socks or mittens or gloves and a hat over the ears
−4 to −1°C or 20-29F	Long-sleeve, medium-weight shirt, another T-shirt, tights and shorts, socks, mittens or gloves, and a hat over the ears
−8 to −3°C or 10-19°F	Long-sleeve, medium-weight shirt, and medium- to heavy-weight shirt, tights and shorts, nylon tracksuit, top and pants, socks, thick mittens, and a hat over the ears
−12 to −7°C or 0-9°F	Two medium- or heavy-weight, long-sleeve tops, thick tights, thick underwear (especially for men), medium to heavy warm-up, gloves and thick mittens, ski mask, a hat over the ears, and Vaseline covering any exposed skin.
−18 to −11°C or −15°F	Two heavy-weight, long-sleeve tops, tights and thick tights, thick underwear (and supporter for men), thick warm-up (top and pants), mittens over gloves, thick ski mask and a hat over ears, Vaseline covering any exposed skin, thicker socks on your feet and other foot protection, as needed
Minus 20 both C & F	Add layers as needed

WHAT NOT TO WEAR

- A heavy coat in winter. If the layer is too thick, you'll heat up, sweat excessively, and cool too much when you take it off.

- White shirt in summer. Sometimes water and perspiration can make white summer fabrics transparent. Colored fabric that holds some of the moisture will give you more of a cooling effect as you run and walk.

- Too much sunscreen – it can interfere with sweating.

- Socks that are too thick in summer. Your feet swell and the pressure from the socks can increase the chance of a black toenail and blisters.

- Lime green shirt with bright pink polka dots (unless you have a lot of confidence and can run fast).

- Cotton in summer is not recommended. The accumulated moisture will be heavy and often chafe.

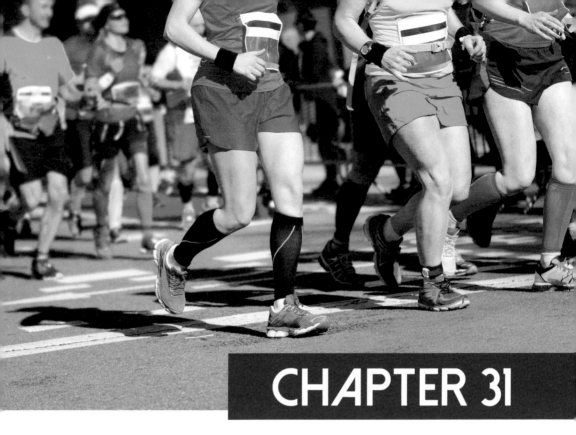

CHAPTER 31

RESOURCES

Group training programs
Galloway training programs, at *www.JeffGalloway.com*

App training programs
lolofit.com – Galloway Ultimat 5K, 10K, and soon, half marathon

Individual coaching
Jeff Galloway as your e-coach: *www.JeffGalloway.com*

Video clips of Jeff's drills, techniques, and training programs for Disney events *www.runDisney.com*

Shoes and clothing: *www.Phidippides.com*

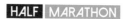

CREDITS

Cover and
interior design: Annika Naas

Layout: www.satzstudio-hilger.de

Cover and
interior photos: © AdobeStock, unless otherwise noted

Editorial
Managing Editor: Elizabeth Evans

MORE GREAT FITNESS BOOKS

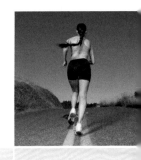

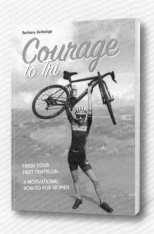

Rutledge

Courage to Tri

Finish Your First Triathlon. A Motivational How-To for Women.

This book is an inspiration and how-to from women who crossed their first finish lines— learning lessons and even changing their lives along the way. It gives women all the tools to master their first triathlon.

256 p., b/w, 50 photos + illus., paperback, 5.5″ x 8.5″
ISBN: 9781782551355
$19.95 US

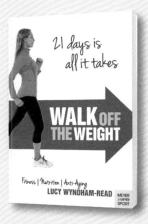

Lucy Wyndham-Read

Walk Off the Weight

Fitness. Nutrition. Anti-Aging.

If you are a walking beginner, an advanced walker, or just like to walk with friends, this is the right book for you. Based on 400 scientific studies, this book is easy to read and gives comprehensive insight into the benefits of Nordic Pole Walking and walking exercise.

168 p., in color, 186 photos, 11 illus., paperback, 6.5" x 9.25"
ISBN 9781782550778
$19.95 US

All information subject to change © Adobe Stock

MEYER & MEYER Sport
Von-Coels-Str. 390
52080 Aachen
Germany

Phone   +49 02 41 - 9 58 10 - 13
Fax   +49 02 41 - 9 58 10 - 10
E-Mail   sales@m-m-sports.com
Website www.m-m-sports.com

MEYER
& MEYER
SPORT

All books available as E-books.

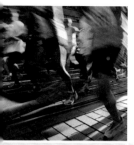

MORE GREAT BOOKS

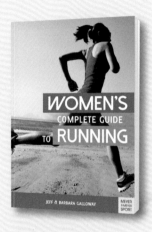

Jeff & Barbara Galloway

Women's Complete Guide to Running

This is the new edition of this comprehensive running guide for women, covering motivation, nutrition, and much more. All the exercises can fit into the busiest lifestyle to relieve stress and enjoy a greater sense of vitality.

4th revised edition, 232 p., in color,
50 photos + illus., paperback, 6.5" x 9.25"
ISBN 9781782551485
$16.95 US

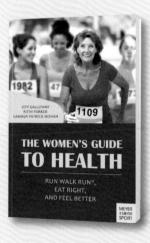

Galloway/Parker/Patrick Mohan

The Women's Guide to Health
Run Walk Run, Eat Right, and Feel Better

This action guide combines Galloway's Run Walk Run programs with the best available medical knowledge for using Run Walk Run and the Mediterranean diet as key treatment modalities for chronic medical conditions related to excess bodyweight.

216 p., b/w, 52 photos, 12 illus., 18 charts,
paperback, 5.5" x 8.5"
ISBN: 9781782551232
$12.95 US

BY JEFF GALLOWAY

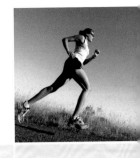

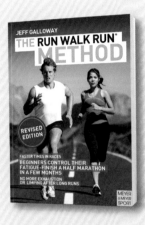

Jeff Galloway

The Run Walk Run Method

Galloway's innovative ideas have opened up the possibility of running and completing a marathon to almost everyone. He believes we were all designed to run and walk, and he keeps finding ways to bring more people into the positive world of exercise.

2nd revised edition, 192 p., in color, 38 photos, 13 charts, paperback, 6.5" x 9.24"
ISBN 9781782550822
$19.95 US

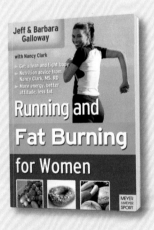

Jeff & Barbara Galloway

Running & Fat Burning for Women

Couch potatoes and seasoned exercisers alike can improve well-being by implementing eating strategies and gentle segments of exercise. Learn about the process of fat depositing and burning and how to gain control over both sides of the issue.

3rd edition, 200 p., in color, 30 photos, paperback, 6.5" x 9.25"
ISBN 9781841262437
$17.95 US

MEYER & MEYER Sport
Von-Coels-Str. 390
52080 Aachen
Germany

Phone   +49 02 41 - 9 58 10 - 13
Fax   +49 02 41 - 9 58 10 - 10
E-Mail   sales@m-m-sports.com
Website   www.m-m-sports.com

MEYER & MEYER SPORT

All books available as E-books.